RECOVERY
A TO Z

D1563270

RECOVERY

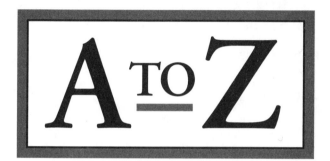

A Handbook of Twelve-Step Key Terms and Phrases

REVISED AND UPDATED

By the Editors of
Central Recovery Press

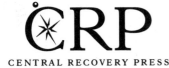

CENTRAL RECOVERY PRESS

CENTRAL RECOVERY PRESS

Central Recovery Press (CRP) is committed to publishing exceptional materials addressing addiction treatment, recovery, and behavioral health care, including original and quality books, audio/visual communications, and web-based new media. Through a diverse selection of titles, it seeks to impact the behavioral health care field with a broad range of unique resources for professionals, recovering individuals and their families, and the general public.

For more information, visit www.centralrecoverypress.com.
Central Recovery Press, Las Vegas, NV 89129
© 2011 by Central Recovery Press, Las Vegas, NV

ISBN-13: 978-1-936290-04-8
ISBN-10: 1-936290-04-9

17 16 15 14 13 12 11   1 2 3 4 5

Publisher: Central Recovery Press
              3371 N Buffalo Drive
              Las Vegas, NV 89129

EDITORS' NOTE: This book is a collection of words and phrases you are likely to hear in the rooms of recovery, including the names of some of the more commonly encountered character defects. We know this is not a definitive or comprehensive listing of these flaws, but we include them in the hope that doing so will help those who are working on their Fourth through Tenth Steps. We welcome your input for inclusion in any future editions.

Cover design and interior by Sara Streifel, Think Creative Design

Thanks to all those in and out of recovery,
especially the clients and staff
of the Las Vegas Recovery Center
who have contributed to the
development of this book.

re·cov·er·y |riˈkəvərē|

CONTENTS

re·cov·er·y |ri'kəvərē|

Preface to the Revised and Updated Edition

Twelve-step programs are simple, but not easy. A newcomer in recovery may feel as if he or she has entered a land where everything—from the customs to the language—is uncomfortably strange. To the ears of a newcomer, twelve-step fellowship members may seem to be speaking in code. This book is intended to help crack that "code" and make twelve-step recovery more accessible and comfortable, to newcomers and their family members alike. Even old timers may learn something new in these pages.

At a time when one's recovery is new, and the old way of life has been abandoned but the new one has not yet firmly taken root, anything that can help smooth the rough edges of anxiety, particularly for a newcomer, may mean the difference between life and death. We hope this book will be one of the tools that will ease the transition into the recovery way of life for you.

The Twelve Steps work. They work so well for those willing to work them, that they have been adapted across numerous fellowships of those suffering from addiction around the world. Whatever the manifestation of addiction, and there are many, the Twelve Steps, wholeheartedly taken with a sponsor and in concert with a recovery fellowship, will work. Whether the manifestation of addiction is food, sex, drugs—including the drug alcohol—gambling, Internet porn, video games, shopping—the Twelve Steps are a widely recognized solution to the insidious disease of addiction. And no matter the fellowship or the specific manifestation, the language in the rooms of recovery is the same. It has been called by many "the language of the heart."

We hope that providing a simple and easy-to-understand reference guide will help you make sense of twelve-step language and help to translate the experience of recovery into a message you can use.

This book may also be of help to your friends and family who are often just as baffled by your newfound recovery life as they were by your active addiction. They knew, perhaps before you knew yourself, that you were on the brink of death, and now, in a relatively short period of time, you are zealously attending meetings every day and becoming engrossed in a healthy and welcome, but equally consuming (and perhaps confusing) way of life, complete with a new vocabulary and new ways of expressing yourself. We know this simple handbook won't solve that problem by itself—sincere and ongoing communication, whatever the words used, will help far more. But we hope this will be a start.

This book can be helpful to those with long-term recovery as they work with newer members, and also can help give the more experienced member a deeper, broader understanding of many of the definitions with which they are already familiar.

This revised and updated edition of *Recovery A to Z* was written with the input and contributions of members of twelve-step recovery programs, and we, the editors of Central Recovery Press, thank them profoundly. This is not meant to be the definitive work on the language of recovery, nor is it written by professionals in recovery or the treatment community. It has, however, been written by those of us who are on the front lines of recovery every day.

The first edition of *Recovery A to Z* was just that—a first edition. In accord with our commitment to keep this handbook as up-to-date as possible based on the input that we have received and changes within the recovery and treatment communities, we offer this revised and updated edition.

Attempting to include all of the ever-changing terminology for every twelve-step fellowship has been a humbling task. There are many different programs and within each program there are myriad slogans, sayings, and phrases. Even within the same community there may not be clear consensus on the meaning of a particular word. We know we have not included every word you may encounter, and we invite you to contact us with corrections, revisions, or new contributions.

One thing you will find in this handbook is a conviction that addiction is one disease with a wide variety of manifestations. Whatever the manifestation, there is no substitute—including this or any book—for attending recovery meetings yourself and finding out what addiction and recovery mean to you.

Research on recovery is ongoing, and science's understanding of the disease of addiction and recovery is ever-evolving. However, for the purposes of this book, when we speak of recovery we are talking about abstinence from alcohol and other drugs or a cessation of addictive behaviors such as compulsive gambling, overeating, shopping, sex, and so on, coupled with active participation in a twelve-step program.

Our heartfelt hope is that you will find this a useful and relevant tool for your own personal recovery.

re·cov·er·y |riˈkəvərē|

Preface to the First Edition

Twelve-step programs have a language of their own. While there are numerous adaptations of the original Twelve Steps, much of the language is the same across all these programs. This dictionary is designed to give those new to twelve-step recovery and friends and family members of persons in recovery, as well as those who have been in the program for a while, a starting point from which they will hopefully develop or expand their own understanding of many of the terms used in meetings and program literature. The words and concepts in this dictionary are specific to the Twelve Steps and many recovery programs. We realize that some of these words and concepts have more general meanings as well.

We hope that providing a simple and easy-to-understand reference guide to help you make sense of the "twelve-step language" will benefit you as you travel along on your journey of recovery.

It also may be of help to friends and family who are often just as baffled by the newfound recovery life of their loved one as they were by that person's active addiction. Their loved one had been on the brink of death, and now, in a relatively short period of time, he or she is zealously attending meetings every day and becoming completely engrossed in a healthy and welcome, but equally consuming (and perhaps confusing) lifestyle, complete with a new vocabulary and new ways of expressing him- or herself. A simple dictionary is not going to solve this problem; sincere and ongoing communication, whatever the words used, will help far more, but again, this is a starting point.

People with some time in the program know better than anyone that understanding and experience changes constantly in recovery. In fact, it is said "the only constant is change." This dictionary can be helpful to those with long-term recovery as they work with newer members, and also can help give the more experienced member a deeper, broader understanding of many of the definitions with which they are familiar.

This dictionary was written with the input and contributions of members of twelve-step recovery programs. It is not meant to be a definitive work on the subject nor is it written by "professionals" in recovery or the treatment community. Instead, it is written by those in recovery for those in recovery.

This first edition is just that—the first. This dictionary will evolve over time just as the members of twelve-step programs do. As more information and feedback is gathered from readers, the more comprehensive the definitions will become. We realize that some words and concepts are missing, and promise that as work on the second edition begins, those words will be added.

Send Us What We Missed

We invite you to send us any words, concepts, or slogans used in your fellowship that weren't included in this handbook. It is our goal to be as clear, authentic, down-to-earth, and comprehensive as possible in order to produce a guide that is accessible to members of all twelve-step fellowships, as well as the general public. This project is truly a work-in-progress.

How to Submit Your Input

USPS/MAIL

Central Recovery Press
Recovery A–Z Submissions
3371 North Buffalo Drive
Las Vegas, NV 89129

EMAIL

CentralRecoveryPress@centralrecovery.com

FAX

(702) 868-5831

FOR OTHER INFORMATION

Visit CentralRecoveryPress.com

Aa

ABSTINENCE and/or ABSTINENT

Free from mind- or mood-altering chemicals or drugs, including the drug alcohol, or addictive behaviors. May be used to refer to a person who is in recovery and who may or may not be actively working the Twelve Steps. Simply to be abstinent—substance-free and/or not engaging in addictive behaviors—is not considered enough for a quality recovery. Working the steps, participating in fellowship meetings, and being of service to others is generally considered "recovery," whereas abstinence simply implies not using or acting out. (See "Dry Drunk.")

Abstinence is also a requirement for successful participation in overcoming compulsive gambling (addiction) in Gamblers Anonymous (GA). The first bet to a problem gambler is comparable to the first drink to an alcoholic or the first hit to a drug addict, and is considered a relapse.

Abstinence in Overeaters Anonymous (OA) is the action of refraining from *compulsive* eating and *compulsive* food behaviors. Since all animals, including humans, must eat in order to live, complete abstinence is obviously not a requirement in this fellowship.

Similarly, members of Sex and Love Addicts Anonymous (SLAA) consider that their recovery does not need to include complete abstinence from romantic relationships and sex, although recovering members may use complete abstinence for short periods of time to gain personal perspective or address a particular issue. In this fellowship, recovery/sobriety is most often defined as adherence to a contract worked out between the sexual/love addict and his or her SLAA sponsor, therapist, or clergy. (See "bottom-line behaviors" for more detailed information.)

ABUSE
Literally, "wrong use," or "bad use." To misuse or mistreat a person or thing. Can refer to an individual's use of legal or street drugs, the drug alcohol, certain compulsive behaviors, or the treatment of one person by another in a relationship (e.g., child abuse, elder abuse). This latter kind of abuse can be verbal, emotional, or physical.

Not all consumption of drugs/medications or alcohol is abusive. Some people can use medications or drink "socially" without abusing these substances. Addicts cannot, period. That is the difference between addicts and non-addicts.

ABUSIVENESS
Viciousness, rudeness, cruelty. To cause physical, emotional, or spiritual injury to another. Considered a character defect.

ACCEPT/ACCEPTANCE
Acknowledge, acquiesce, recognize/recognition, acknowledgement. Considered a spiritual principle meaning to recognize and/or resign oneself to a situation, occurrence, truth, fact, etc. To accept a fact does not imply that one agrees with or is happy with it.

ACOA
Adult Children of Alcoholics. Sometimes used to refer to a person who is the offspring of an alcoholic; other times refers to Al-Anon meetings specifically for ACOAs.

ACCOUNTABILITY/ACCOUNTABLE
Answerability/answerable, responsibility/responsible. In recovery terms, being accountable means to honor one's word. Answering to another individual about personal actions, behaviors, thoughts, or feelings. Considered a spiritual principle.

ACTING OUT

Acting out is not the same as "acting up," although many use the terms interchangeably without knowing the difference. Acting out is an unconscious ego defense mechanism. Without being aware of it, persons who act out engage in some kind of behavior that (temporarily) eases the emotional pain and anxiety caused by an entirely unconscious conflict between their instincts and their conscience. Acting up is simply bad behavior.

In sex-addiction recovery, "acting out" is the result of the failure to exert control over or intervene on one's sexual behavior. There is no particular sexual behavior that constitutes sexual addiction; it is in the relationship between sexual feelings and activities and a person's total life experience that sex addiction exists.

ACTION

Deed, feat, movement. Task undertaken in order to achieve an outcome. Action implies putting effort into a thought or decision. When the word "action" is used in recovery, it could mean staying clean/sober/ in recovery/abstinent, attending meetings, talking and working with a sponsor, writing on the steps or doing step work, service work, changing behavior, etc.

ACTIVE ADDICTION

The time in an individual's life when he or she actively used mind- or mood-altering chemicals/drugs, including the drug alcohol, or participated in a destructive behavior such as compulsive gambling, overeating, or the unhealthy use of sex or love. Also refers to the time period prior to getting clean/sober/in recovery/abstinent, when a person's addiction was active.

ADDICT

A person with a physical, mental, emotional, and spiritual reaction to the use of mind- or mood-altering chemicals and/or certain behaviors; one who is dependent upon a substance or behavior. A person who has the disease of addiction. A person who uses excessive amounts of any number of substances or participates in excessive behaviors that may be considered destructive to the self, which may include, but are not limited to, drugs, alcohol, food, sex, gambling, spending money, shopping, video games, or pornography. Characterized as being obsessive and compulsive. A term for a recovering member of certain twelve-step programs.

ADDICTION

Dependence, craving, habit. A chronic brain disease that affects a person physically, mentally, emotionally, and spiritually. Addiction is obsessive thoughts, followed by compulsive behaviors that result in a self-centered attitude and pursuit of one's own immediate desires. Denial makes detection and identification of addiction all the more difficult and obstructs treatment and ongoing recovery.

Addiction usually results from an unhealthy and mood-altering relationship between a person and the manifestations(s) of his or her addiction, whether *substances*—drugs that can be used to change how a person feels, regardless of whether these drugs come from the street (cocaine/crack, heroin/opiates, meth/speed, marijuana, hallucinogens) or are prescribed by a doctor (painkillers, tranquilizers, sedatives) or are bought at a store (alcohol, over-the-counter medications, and other substances, such as inhalants) or *activities* such as gambling, eating, shopping/spending, sex, pornography, Internet use, video gaming, love/relationships, etc.—to the point where using the substance or engaging in the activity becomes beyond voluntary control and continues regardless of increasingly negative consequences.

Addiction affects people regardless of ethnicity, age, gender, sexual orientation, religious affiliation, economic standing, intellect, education, family environment, etc.

ADMITTED/ADMISSION

Disclosed, acknowledged, confessed. Acknowledgment of a fact or truth. In recovery terms, to admit means to acknowledge that one is powerless over addiction, that his or her life is unmanageable, and that recovery is possible. Many twelve-step programs list the substance or particular behavior over which a person is powerless in their First Step (such as addiction, alcohol, cocaine, gambling, etc.). Admission of the problem is the first step that must be taken before someone can get and stay clean/sober/in recovery/abstinent and grow in his or her own personal recovery.

ADULT CHILDREN OF ALCOHOLICS (ACOA)

A twelve-step program of women and men who grew up in alcoholic or otherwise dysfunctional homes. "Adult Child" is used sometimes to refer to a person who is the offspring of an alcoholic. Members look at how their childhood affected them in the past and influences them in the present. This is referred to as "The Problem." "The Solution" is how members learn to accept a loving higher power of their understanding and find freedom from the past and a way to improve their lives today.

ADVICE/ADVISE

Counsel, recommendations, suggestions. To give another person one's opinion or recommendation regarding the action that person should take in a situation or circumstance. Can be negative when unsolicited or not based on the personal experience of the advisor. Opposite of sharing one's experience, strength, and hope, which is considered the foundation of twelve-step support.

AFFILIATED

Joined, united, allied. Associated or connected to a group, business, facility, center, organization, etc. To be known publicly to be associated with a group, business, or organization. Affiliation can be direct or implied. Twelve-step programs are not affiliated, as stated in Tradition Six, with other professional organizations, treatment centers, recovery homes, or government agencies even if twelve-step meetings are held in such facilities.

AFTERCARE

Continuing services or follow-up care offered by many inpatient addiction treatment and rehabilitation programs for patients who attended or resided at the facility. These programs often require "graduates" to attend continuing sessions for a pre-determined length of time. Some of the topics covered in aftercare address reentry into society, employment issues, relapse prevention, and other recovery-related topics. Participation in aftercare is not the same as twelve-step meeting and fellowship participation.

AGGRESSION

Force, insistence, belligerence. (At odds with calm, serenity.) Cause of behaving in a hostile, overly intense, or harsh manner. Considered a character defect. **Note:** One can be assertive without being aggressive.

AGNOSTIC

Disbeliever, doubter, nonbeliever. Agnosticism is the intellectual position that the existence of God or other spiritual beings is uncertain or unknowable. An agnostic may believe there is a higher power of sorts, but does not believe in a traditional concept of God. The steps are not dependent on this belief and many agnostics can and do develop their own understanding of a higher power and benefit from working the Twelve Steps.

AL-ANON

A fellowship whose members share their own experience, strength, and hope with each other to learn a better way of life and to find happiness whether their alcoholic loved one is still drinking or not. Al-Anon's program of recovery is based on the Twelve Steps and Twelve Traditions of Alcoholics Anonymous.

ALATEEN

A twelve-step fellowship of young Al-Anon members, usually teenagers, whose lives have been affected by someone else's drinking. Alateen groups are typically sponsored by Al-Anon members.

ALCOHOL

Ethyl alcohol (ETOH) or ethanol produced by distillation or brewing. Consumed as a liquid (beer, wine, or spirits), it is a central nervous system depressant which, when consumed in large quantities, impairs motor skills, judgment, and brain function. It is a drug and is potentially addictive; consumption causes intoxication and when consumed in large quantities and/or over time can lead to death.

ALCOHOLIC

A person with the disease of addiction manifested by the excessive consumption of alcohol (beer, wine, spirits) and who has an unhealthy relationship to alcohol. One whose life is adversely affected by his or her consumption of alcohol. Of a substance, relates to whether or not it contains alcohol. A term for a recovering member of the twelve-step program of Alcoholics Anonymous.

ALCOHOLICS ANONYMOUS (AA)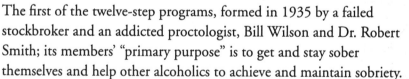

The first of the twelve-step programs, formed in 1935 by a failed stockbroker and an addicted proctologist, Bill Wilson and Dr. Robert Smith; its members' "primary purpose" is to get and stay sober themselves and help other alcoholics to achieve and maintain sobriety. A fellowship or society for people with the disease of alcoholism.

AA owns the copyright to the Twelve Steps of Alcoholics Anonymous and has the authority to allow other fellowships to reprint them through express permission. *Alcoholics Anonymous* is the official name of the primary text used in the fellowship of AA. It was written by Bill Wilson and others.

ALCOHOLISM

A chronic, progressive, and fatal disease that manifests as a reaction in the body to alcohol and a physical, mental, emotional, and spiritual need for alcohol. An alcoholic is said to suffer from and to live with the disease of alcoholism.

ALIENATE

Estrange, disaffect, set against. To separate from others. To create distance or isolation; may be done consciously or unconsciously, so as to conceal behaviors that may not be accepted by others and to continue to engage in such behaviors. To withdraw from others or to be unresponsive to them. Alienation is often considered a character defect.

ALTERNATE DELEGATE (AD)

A person elected by a regional service committee. This is a learning or training position. The AD will eventually assume the regional delegate (RD) position and carry the regional conscience on specific topics and/ or motions to the service conferences of various fellowships. Some of the twelve-step programs that have alternate and regional delegates include Narcotics Anonymous, Alcoholics Anonymous, and Overeaters Anonymous. This is terminology specific to the service structure found in many twelve-step fellowships.

AMENDS

Atonements, reparations, compensations. A key part of the twelve-step process, particularly Steps Eight and Nine. To make amends is to express contrition for and correct an old wrong or change a behavior that has harmed others. Amends may include a request for forgiveness for prior actions that may have harmed an individual or group. May be direct, as in paying back money stolen or borrowed, or indirect, in cases where it would be imprudent or impossible (for example, when the injured party has died). These indirect amends are often referred to as "ongoing amends" or "living amends," which consist of a continuing and deliberate effort to refrain from repeating a behavior that caused harm to another person or group.

ANGER

Fury, rage, antagonism. Anger is an emotional response to a real or imagined "wrong," injustice, or frustration in the present. It is a normal, natural emotion that, in many situations is a healthy and appropriate response. Problems with anger usually occur in how this powerful feeling is expressed. Anger can be expressed along a wide range—from suppressing it (i.e., not expressing it outwardly, keeping it inside to the point where a person may not even be aware that he or she is angry) all the way to exploding, which can include screaming, verbal abuse, property damage, and even physical violence. When expressed in these ways, anger is considered a character defect.

In most circumstances, anger is really a secondary emotion. It often forms immediately and automatically (this happens unconsciously so there may be no awareness of it) in response to something that or someone who brings up feelings of hurt, fear, and/or inadequacy. When most people experience these primary emotions, they feel vulnerable, and their energy and attention are focused internally. This inward focus on one's own vulnerabilities is extremely uncomfortable, especially for people who are used to focusing on other people and things outside of themselves.

ANONYMITY

Namelessness, obscurity, vagueness. The state of being unknown, unidentified. A spiritual principle that serves several purposes in recovery, including:

* Promotion of the ideal of humility by helping ensure that all persons in recovery are equal, with no member greater or lesser than another.

* Protection of a person's identity by not referring to them outside of a group or meeting setting. Since addiction is still poorly understood outside of the recovery community and many, even some of those who are new to the programs, consider it a moral failing rather than a disease, anonymity is often necessary to protect the jobs and reputations of those seeking recovery.

ANONYMOUS
Unidentified, unknown, unnamed. (See Anonymity.)

ANOREXIA NERVOSA
An eating disorder that causes the victim to drastically reduce his or her food intake to the point of becoming dangerously malnourished and underweight. Anorexia nervosa is the opposite of compulsive overeating and is considered a psychological disorder that is often accompanied by excessive exercising, taking laxatives and diuretics, and/or taking diet pills in order to maintain a thin body. Research has shown that anorexia nervosa is similar to any type of manifestation of addiction.

ANOREXIC, SEXUAL
In sex-and-love- or relationship-recovery terms, sexual anorexia refers to an unhealthy withdrawal from participation in relationships or sexual activity or other forms of physical engagement with others. This is different from a self-imposed period of abstinence from relationships and sex, which is undertaken in order for the addict to gain perspective.

Sexual anorexia can manifest in a variety of forms, including isolation, keeping oneself too busy to date or participate in relationships with others, or through pursing relationships with unavailable people.

ANOREXICS AND BULIMICS ANONYMOUS (ABA)
A twelve-step fellowship for individuals that helps members to maintain sobriety in their eating practices. ABA considers eating disorders to be about an illusion of control over food and body weight and defines "sobriety" as surrender of this illusion of control to a higher power. The only requirement for membership in ABA is a desire to stop unhealthy eating practices.

ANXIETY

Nervousness, unease, apprehension. A feeling of being overwhelmed and/or overly concerned/worried by circumstances that may or may not be within one's control. Anxiety is often focused on events/circumstances that have not yet happened. A form of fear.

APATHY

Lethargy, indifference, lack of concern. Lacking interest in something or someone. To be indifferent to either one's own or another's feelings, experiences, or circumstances. Can be a symptom of depression. To have apathy toward others in recovery or toward the Twelve Steps can often lead to relapse.

APPRAISAL

Evaluation, assessment, review. To look at oneself either through writing or sharing with a sponsor or support group. Usually done through an inventory or step work.

APPROPRIATE

Apt, correct, proper. Behavior or language that fits a given setting. Behaving in a way that is acceptable to another person, group, or society. Appropriate meeting behavior may be learned through the example of others at twelve-step meetings.

APPROVAL SEEKING

Behavior geared toward obtaining the goodwill of another person or group. Needing, wanting, or depending upon validation from another person to make one feel better about him- or herself, sometimes at the expense of one's own genuine wants or needs.

AREA SERVICE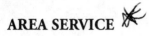

A committee meeting usually held monthly in which volunteer group service representatives (GSRs), subcommittee chairpersons, and administration members meet to discuss area issues; vote on motions affecting groups, the area, region, and world services of the fellowship; distribute literature; collect Seventh Tradition donations; and offer assistance to groups, etc. This is terminology specific to the service structure found in most twelve-step fellowships.

ARROGANCE

Egotism, self-importance, cockiness. Feeling or acting superior to others. Lacking humility about one's possessions, talents, gifts, or abilities, and using them as a means of making other people feel inferior or "less-than." Considered a character defect.

ASSETS

Possessions, belongings, property/worldly goods. May be material or abstract, such as positive character attributes and aspects. Character traits or strengths that benefit recovery and the lives of others. May be referred to as part of a Fourth Step inventory process. Part of having humility is being aware of one's assets as well as one's liabilities.

ASSUME

Presuppose, guess, imagine. To take a thing, person, situation, etc. for granted without proper investigation or knowledge of all the information pertaining to that thing, person, or situation. Assumptions may lead to resentments when one person takes for granted that another will behave in a certain way, but that person does not.

ATHEIST(S) ✗

Nonbeliever(s). Active or passive disbelief or non-belief in the existence of a God or gods. People who do not believe in a higher power that is a god(s), deity, or deities. Atheists who are in twelve-step recovery may believe their higher power or "power greater than" is anything from the Twelve Steps, to their higher self, to the group, or anything non-material that is positive, uplifting, and greater than themselves. As proven by the number of atheists in recovery today, one does not have to believe in a god in order to find and stay in recovery.

ATMOSPHERE

Mood, ambiance, environment; as in "atmosphere of recovery." An environment that is conducive to open and honest sharing and that allows the message of recovery to be heard. An atmosphere of recovery allows those in recovery to feel that they are safe, even temporarily, from active addiction. Referred to in relation to a group or meeting's tone or environment.

ATTACHMENT

Connection, affection, bond. To have a connection to a person, place, thing, or outcome (may be positive or negative).

ATTENTION SEEKING

Similar to approval seeking; except that the attention sought may be either negative or positive. May be expressed in actions or words.

ATTITUDE

Outlook, approach, mindset. State of mind or belief that is reflected in one's actions. In recovery, a positive or negative mindset and manner of acting that is usually a direct result of one's spiritual fitness achieved through practice of the Twelve Steps.

ATTRACTION

Pull, magnetism, appeal. A strong desire for something because of its appearance, attitude, or other appealing qualities. Twelve-step programs do not advertise or recruit; their appeal to potential members is assumed to be based on the inherent attractiveness of a life lived in recovery as opposed to the slow death of active addiction. Is found in the Eleventh Tradition of twelve-step programs, which states ". . . public relations policy is based on attraction rather than promotion . . . ."

AUTONOMY

Self-rule, self-government, independence. Able to make one's own decisions. To be able to govern as one wishes without outside direction, interference, or involvement. Acting in one's own interest. Also refers to Tradition Four in which "each group is autonomous." This tradition cautions that while groups may be autonomous, they need to ensure that their actions do not affect the fellowship as a whole.

AWAKENING

Developing, beginning, stirring. The mental adjustment or spiritual awakening necessary for long-term recovery from addiction is said to come about as "the result" of working all of the Twelve Steps; however, in the beginning, simply awakening to one's problem is enough to allow a person to enter recovery and begin working Step One.

AWARENESS

Alertness, consciousness, attentiveness. A realization of truth in regard to some situation, idea, attitude, or behavior. Considered the first part in the process of change; something one must have or be open to having before being able to address addiction.

AWFULIZING

Exaggerating the difficulties associated with many life experiences. Always seeing the worst in any given situation. A form of distorted thinking in recovery that may lead to relapse.

AWOL GROUPS

A Way of Life (AWOL) groups are closed groups of overeaters, formed for the sole purpose of working the Twelve Steps; not, strictly speaking, Overeaters Anonymous (OA) groups. However, many OA members do attend AWOL groups for additional support.

Bb

BAGGAGE

Casual term for unresolved past issues brought into present situations and current events. Fears, insecurities, and past harms that become ingrained into an individual's psychological makeup and that influence his or her automatic responses to situations. May also be referred to as "the wreckage of our past."

BALANCE

Stability, equilibrium, steadiness. A quality that allows for coping with all areas of life in equal proportion and devoting an equal amount of time, effort, and concern to each area. Some areas commonly considered are work, emotional, mental, and physical health, spiritual well-being, and extracurricular activities or leisure.

BASIC TEXT

Another name for the primary textbook of the twelve-step program of Narcotics Anonymous. The actual title for the Basic Text is *Narcotics Anonymous*. A recovery text written over a number of years by committees comprised of recovering addicts and designed to articulate the philosophy and approach of the NA program. Also includes personal stories from recovering addicts. It was first published in 1983. There have been six subsequent editions released since then.

BASICS

Essentials, fundamentals, nuts-and-bolts. Program slang that refers to the fundamental or central actions one must take when entering a twelve-step program, which include but are not limited to attending meetings, getting a sponsor, working steps, and being of service to others both inside and out of one's fellowship/program.

BEGINNER

Novice, learner, apprentice. Also referred to as a newcomer, a person new to the recovery process or one returning from a relapse. There is no commonly agreed-upon time frame for how long a person remains a newcomer or beginner, but newcomer status usually relates more to chronological time in recovery, not in the number of steps one has worked.

BEHAVIOR

Deeds, manners, conduct. Behaviors can indicate a person's progress in recovery or lack thereof; can indicate a state of mind when words sometimes do not. Some behaviors advance recovery, others impede it; especially "old" behaviors that recall or might trigger a return to active addiction.

BELIEF

Faith, conviction, principle; trust. A strongly held idea or concept; part of one's value system. The way a person or group views a concept or idea. Confidence in an idea, a person, a group, or a higher power.

BETRAYAL/BETRAYING

A violation of another's trust; letting someone down; to deceive or misguide. Being false or disloyal to. Breaking faith with another. Considered a character defect.

BIG BOOK

The primary text of the twelve-step program of Alcoholics Anonymous. The complete original title was *Alcoholics Anonymous: The Story of How Many Thousands of Men and Women Have Recovered from Alcoholism;* it was first published in 1939 with four subsequent editions published since.

The primary author of the Big Book was Bill Wilson; contributors included Dr. Robert Smith—together these two men ("Bill W" and "Dr. Bob"), are considered the co-founders of Alcoholics Anonymous. Other early contributors to the book included Dr. William Silkworth, the "little doctor who loved drunks," though he himself was not one.

BLACKOUT/BLACK OUT

As a noun, a loss of memory due to consuming excessive amounts of alcohol and/or other drugs; particularly associated with alcohol abuse and intoxication. Abusers of alcohol or alcoholics will often speak of having little or no memory of certain events because of being blacked out, or "in a blackout."

To "black out" is not, as is sometimes thought, to "pass out" or to lose consciousness—this dangerous condition, blackout—when one can walk, talk, and drive a vehicle—is an altered state of consciousness. Many alcoholics have "come out of a blackout" to find themselves married to a complete stranger, in a hospital bed with broken limbs or worse, under arrest for brawling or assault, or even for having killed a person or persons while driving under the influence.

BODY DYSMORPHIC DISORDER

Body dysmorphic disorder is defined as a "somatoform disorder" marked by a preoccupation with an *imagined* defect in the sufferer's appearance that causes significant distress or impairment in various areas of life. For example, if the problem is weight-related, the individual may develop an eating disorder that can be treated with twelve-step support.

BOREDOM

Monotony, tedium, world-weariness. A feeling that time is passing too slowly because there is nothing stimulating to occupy one's attention. Feeling disinterested in current activities, unable to generate interest in or motivation to start new activities. May be the result of not having a hobby or interest in positive activities. Sometimes a symptom of depression.

Newcomers occasionally confuse the tranquility of life in recovery with "boredom" until they become accustomed to living without the drama and crises of active addiction.

BOTTOM LINE(S)

In sexual- or relationship-addiction recovery "bottom-line" behavior is behavior that is considered off-limits or not in line with one's recovery. Bottom lines are usually determined with the assistance of a sponsor (in SA or SLAA, for example) and often in conjunction with a First Step. Bottom lines may include such activities as masturbation, having sex outside one's committed relationship, or engaging in other sexual intrigue. (See also Inner-, Middle-, and Outer-Circle Behaviors.)

BOUNDARIES

Borders, limits, margins. May refer to limitations, rules, or expectations of personal space, allowing others to know what is and is not acceptable in a relationship. Properly set and maintained, boundaries can protect a person. The goal of many relationship-based twelve-step programs is to set and maintain effective and healthy boundaries.

BUGABOOS

An imaginary "something" that instills or causes fear, annoyance, or trouble in a person. Old feelings, ideas, concepts, or thought processes that may resurface, particularly in relation to feelings of inadequacy or insecurities about the ability to grow, change, or experience feelings of happiness or freedom.

BULIMIA NERVOSA

Bulimia nervosa is a serious, potentially life-threatening eating disorder, related to anorexia nervosa and compulsive overeating, with certain differences. People with bulimia nervosa may binge and purge, eating large amounts of food and then trying to get rid of the extra calories in an unhealthy way. Bulimia is classified in two ways:

• Purging bulimia: Regularly engaging in self-induced vomiting or the misuse of laxatives, diuretics, or enemas to compensate for binges.

• Nonpurging bulimia: Regular use of other methods to rid oneself of calories and prevent weight gain, such as fasting or over-exercising.

Cc

CAME (as in TO BELIEVE) ➡

Moved toward, arrived, occurred to the mind. In twelve-step programs, "came to believe" is a phrase in the Second Step that refers to the developing belief in a power outside of oneself that can help one to recover. This is something that may not happen instantly, but rather over time and through examples of that power's presence in one's life.

CARE/CARING

Concern, thoughtfulness; nurturing, protecting. To have and show concern for someone or something else by taking a personal interest in his or her well-being. May also relate to self-care, which would include taking appropriate action to maintain recovery, as in "to care for one's own recovery."

CARETAKING

In recovery terms, "caretaking" means taking inappropriate responsibility for the feelings, thoughts, behaviors, problems, choices, and lives of others. Related to codependence and enabling. Codependent caretaking often can make one feel victimized and used. Al-Anon, Nar-Anon, and CoDA are twelve-step programs that can help persons recover from unhealthy caretaking.

CARRY (IT OUT)

As in, ". . . the power to carry it out" in Step Eleven. "Carry it out" refers to doing the will of one's higher power rather than seeking to follow one's own will.

CARRY (THE MESSAGE)

Transmit, move, pass on. The message is that recovery is possible; sharing one's experience with the Twelve Steps is "carrying the message," conveying the idea that practicing the Twelve Steps is an effective way to find recovery from addiction.

CHANGE

Modify, alter, transform. Becoming different or transforming through a process of working the Twelve Steps, going to meetings, listening to feedback from those with experience, and helping others do the same thing. A process of discovering the root of certain behaviors that have caused harm and finding new and healthy behaviors to replace them. A fundamental concept in twelve-step programs.

CHARACTER

Temperament, personality, the nature of a thing or person. The character of a person is often developed from personal and environmental experiences. In recovery terms, an individual's character can be repaired through working the Twelve Steps. Step Six refers to character defects that if not addressed can set the stage for relapse.

CHARACTER DEFECTS

Flaws, imperfections, shortcomings. Personality traits that are considered negative and/or behaviors that cause damage to self or others. Character defects may mask deeper issues that need to be addressed if one is to stay in the recovery process. Not to be confused with mere negative thoughts or feelings; character defects are the personal negative elements that are at the root of maladaptive actions and behaviors. There is no shame in possessing character defects, as they are part of human nature. The shame is in acting on them instead of working steps and asking a higher power to remove those defects that stand in the way of one's recovery.

As related to recovery, character defects are typically discovered through writing a Fourth Step inventory and sharing that inventory in the Fifth Step. Character defects are addressed specifically in Steps Six and Seven.

CHARACTERISTIC

Quality, trait, attribute. Typical of a person or thing, distinguishing him or her or it from other people or things.

CHRONIC PAIN

Physical distress, discomfort, or a pain/ache/soreness that lasts for longer than six months and is usually the result of illness, injury, or trauma, although the cause may sometimes be unknown. Chronic pain is often classified as an illness in itself, emotional, as well as physical. It is frequently treated with medications that under other circumstances might constitute a relapse or which might cause addiction.

CIRCUIT SPEAKER

A circuit speaker is a program member with a gift for public speaking and a charismatic way of "pitching" his or her experience in recovery. They travel at the invitation of local groups and may speak all across the country and around the world.

Some circuit speakers become so sought after or venerated, problems of ego and hero-worship can arise; additionally, some members feel that circuit speakers can sound "stale" or "canned" after telling their story so many times. However, many a newcomer has been inspired by a circuit speaker, and hearing a speaker with an entertaining or inspiring story may be just what a newcomer or other member needs to stay in recovery for one more day.

CLEAN

Unsoiled, spotless, dirt-free. In recovery terms, to be abstinent from all mind- and mood-altering chemicals with the purpose of recovering from addiction. Maintaining abstinence from a particular addictive behavior with the purpose of recovering from that particular manifestation of addiction.

CLEAN TIME

The amount of time a person has abstained from the use of drugs, including the drug alcohol, or addictive behavior. The term *sobriety* is used in Alcoholics Anonymous to describe an individual's continual abstinence and participation in the program. Clean time is the preferred expression used in Narcotics Anonymous.

CLOSED MEETING

A twelve-step meeting that is only open to those who identify as suffering from the substance or behavior the meeting's fellowship addresses; e.g., a closed NA meeting is only for drug addicts; a closed AA meeting is for alcoholics; and a closed GA meeting is only for compulsive gamblers. (A person who is in the process of questioning whether he or she has the disease of addiction may attend a closed meeting, but only alcoholics, addicts, or compulsive gamblers may share at these meetings.)

Any member of the public who wants information about any of these fellowships can attend open meetings where all are welcome. Open meetings of many fellowships can generally be found in local directories.

CLOSED-MINDED

Narrow-minded, insular, unreceptive. The opposite of open-minded. Rigidly disinclined to consider new ideas or concepts; clinging to already-established beliefs.

CLUTTERERS ANONYMOUS (CLA)

Clutterers Anonymous is a twelve-step fellowship for individuals for whom hoarding/cluttering has become a compulsion. Clutterers Anonymous defines the need to fill one's home/life with possessions as an expression of an inner or spiritual emptiness that the clutterer compulsively tries to fill by clinging to "useless objects, non-productive ideas, meaningless activities, and unsatisfying relationships" much as any addict seeks to fix emotional pain with chemicals or self-destructive behaviors.

COCAINE ANONYMOUS (CA)

A twelve-step fellowship for individuals who are addicted to cocaine, including "crack" cocaine. The only requirement for membership is a desire to stop using cocaine.

Cocaine Anonymous began in Los Angeles in 1982 with its first meeting being held in Hollywood, California. CA has since expanded throughout the United States and Canada with approximately 2,000 meetings being held in the US. There are roughly 175 meeting now being held in Europe. The fellowship's recovery text is *Hope, Faith & Courage: Stories from the Fellowship of Cocaine Anonymous* and was published in 1994.

CODEPENDENT/CODEPENDENCY

Mutually reliant/needy; relating to a partnership in which one (or both) member(s) is (are) unhealthily psychologically reliant on the other. One who is involved in such a relationship may be called "a codependent." There is a twelve-step program for codependents called CoDA.

CODEPENDENTS ANONYMOUS (CoDA)

A twelve-step fellowship whose primary focus is to help people develop healthy relationships. The only requirement for membership is a desire for healthy and loving relationships. Its recovery text is called *Co-Dependents Anonymous*.

CoDA was founded in 1986 in Phoenix, Arizona and has meetings in more than forty countries with approximately 1,200 meetings in the US.

CODEPENDENTS OF SEX ADDICTS (COSA)

A twelve-step recovery program for men and women whose lives have been affected by another person's compulsive sexual behavior. COSA is a separate fellowship from Sex Addicts Anonymous (SAA), but cooperates with SAA.

COLLAPSE

Crumple, fall down, disintegrate. Also refers to having a breakdown of a mental, physical, emotional, or spiritual nature. May manifest as exhaustion, illness, or emotional outbursts such as extended bouts of crying or fits of rage. A mental, emotional, and/or spiritual collapse may be painful, but also can lead to a breakthrough that may be needed in recovery.

COMMITMENT

Vow, promise, pledge. An agreement to perform a certain task, job, or function or to fulfill a certain role or responsibility, possibly recurring over a specified period of time. Often used in reference to the various positions found in the service structure of many twelve-step programs, as in a "service commitment."

COMMITTEE

Group, board, team. A steering or business group comprised of fellowship members charged with carrying out the needed business functions of the group, or with carrying out specified task(s), such as organizing or directing another group, or fulfilling a stated mission. A group accountable to another body or group of people. This is terminology specific to the service structure found in most twelve-step fellowships.

Some members will talk about the "committee" going on in their heads. This is a light-hearted reference to the negative self-talk many in recovery often engage in.

COMMON BOND

Mutual union, attachment, camaraderie. The connection among members of a twelve-step fellowship is the shared disease of addiction, and the reason people come together at meetings is for the common solution and common bond they find in recovery.

COMMON NEEDS MEETINGS

Meetings that are specifically designed for people in recovery with other issues in common such as their gender, sexual orientation, notoriety/celebrity, profession, age, etc.

COMMON SENSE

Coherent, sound, rational thought. Reasonable and practical judgment based on experience rather than study. Instinctual thoughts or ideas about a given situation or how to react to events. Considered to be natural knowingness.

COMMON WELFARE

From the First Tradition of twelve-step programs; refers to the collective well-being of the fellowship and the reciprocal support needed in order for the fellowship to thrive. In other words, members could not find and/or stay in recovery if the fellowship were not in existence and the fellowship could not exist without its members.

COMMUNICATION

A message, announcement, or transmission. The practice of ensuring that both parties in a relationship understand each other by talking or writing with the intention of conveying a thought, feeling, idea, opinion, answer, directive, or request. A verbal or non-verbal expression of one's thoughts that may include sign language, facial expressions, body posturing, etc. It is considered an essential part of relationships and necessary for forming healthy bonds and/or intimacy with others.

COMPASSION

Care, concern, kindness. Having or displaying love or concern for another or toward oneself through words or actions. Showing consideration for another's well-being. Being sensitive to what another might be feeling. Having tenderness or being gentle with another and conscious of the impact of one's actions on another. Considered a spiritual principle.

COMPETITIVENESS

Vying with others for victory, having a sense of rivalry, striving to outdo another. Desiring one's own success above all else.

COMPLACENCY

Stagnation, smugness, apathy. Being satisfied with matters as they are while ignoring their negative aspects. Being stuck in a rut or situation without taking any action to do anything about it. Dangerous in recovery if the recovery process ceases or stagnates and the disease of addiction starts to gain more ground in the thought processes or actions of the individual.

COMPLAINING

Whiny, belligerent, irritable. Expressing feelings of pain, discomfort, or resentment. Making a formal accusation or bringing a formal charge. Considered a character defect.

COMPLIANCE

Conformity (with rules), obedience, observance of rules. Usually a term used in treatment or clinical settings that refers to abiding by or agreeing with a particular facility's rules, regulations, requests, and/or directives.

COMPULSION

Urge, impulse, craving. The uncontrollable need to act in a particular manner, even with the knowledge it will be harmful, is a major component of the disease of addiction.

Compulsions are actions that spring from obsessions (thoughts); e.g., a person with an obsession about dirt and germs might try to relieve that obsession by repeated hand-washing. The obsession is dirt; the compulsion is hand-washing.

CONCEPTS (as in TWELVE CONCEPTS)
In recovery terms, the "concepts" refer to the ideals and suggested ways to perform service work in a healthy and recovery-oriented manner. Many twelve-step programs have incorporated the Twelve Concepts into their service structure. Some examples include The Twelve Concepts of NA Service (Narcotics Anonymous), The Twelve Concepts for World Service (Alcoholics Anonymous), The Twelve Concepts for OA Service (Overeaters Anonymous), and The Twelve Concepts of Service (Al-Anon/Alateen). This is terminology specific to the service structure found in most twelve-step fellowships.

CONCERN
Worry, apprehension, alarm. To have or show a positive regard for someone or something. Can be positive in nature when an individual is being empathetic or helping one in his or her recovery; similar to compassion. On the negative side, can turn into worry, fretting, or anxiety over a situation or person because of a lack of knowledge about the outcome and inability to trust in a higher power.

CONDITIONAL
Provisional, qualified; within limits. Dependent on certain situations or circumstances. The love of a higher power is said to be unconditional.

CONFERENCE

Meeting, forum, discussion. Usually refers to business meetings that are held annually or biennially to make decisions regarding the literature of twelve-step programs/fellowships, discuss concerns or issues within the fellowship, elect board members/trustees, conduct fellowship business, and serve as a decision-making body of the collective group conscience of the fellowship. These conferences are usually composed of representatives (delegates) from states, regions, and/or countries, depending on the fellowship/program. Some examples include World Service Conference of Narcotics Anonymous, the General Service Conference of Alcoholics Anonymous, the World Service Business Conference of Overeaters Anonymous, Nicotine Anonymous World Services Conference, and Debtors Anonymous World Service Conference. This is terminology specific to the service structure found in many twelve-step fellowships.

CONFERENCE AGENDA REPORT (CAR)

Most common usage is found in Narcotics Anonymous; however, other twelve-step programs do generate a conference agenda for their service business meetings/conferences. A report sent out to membership groups of Narcotics Anonymous. The report lists all motions and discussions to be approved by the NA fellowship as a whole, including many recovery literature projects. This is terminology specific to the service structure found in some twelve-step fellowships.

CONFERENCE-APPROVED LITERATURE

Printed material (books, pamphlets, or booklets) used in meetings and published or approved by the international or national service body of the twelve-step fellowship to which it applies. Material that is not approved by the conference (or fellowship) is not distributed at the fellowship's meetings. Books and materials written by other organizations are generally not sold or used in twelve-step meetings; however, there are many fine books and other recovery materials usually sold as "self-help books," that while not "conference-approved literature," have nevertheless helped numerous addicts.

CONFIDENCE

Poise, assurance, belief in oneself. An assuredness or self-confidence that usually accompanies or is the result of working the Twelve Steps. Unquestioning faith or trust in the ability of an individual, group, idea, or concept, often due to personal experience, observation, or reputation.

CONFIDENTIALITY

Discretion, privacy, prudence. The practice of keeping private matters and/or issues secure or safe. Assurance that personal information is not shared with those it does not concern. Confidentiality is to be expected from a counselor, sponsor, confidant, or friend.

CONFLICT

Clash, disagreement, contradiction. The inability to come to an agreement or make a decision. As related to recovery, many twelve-step programs believe that the spiritual principles embodied in the steps are never in conflict.

CONFRONT

Face (as in come face-to-face with a person or situation), meet head-on, challenge. To tell someone something he or she may not want to hear about him- or herself and/or his or her behavior. Also refers to issues/situations a person must address in order to move forward in recovery.

CONFUSION

Perplexity, puzzlement, bewilderment. A state of uncertainty, feeling lost, being mystified, lacking a clear understanding; being overwhelmed with too much information.

CONSCIENCE (See GROUP CONSCIENCE)

Scruples, having a sense of moral awareness of right and wrong, ethics. Conscience constrains behavior, compelling individuals to act in certain (principled, ethical) ways and refrain from behavior that is unprincipled or unethical or that may cause harm.

CONSCIOUS (CONSCIOUS CONTACT)

Cognizant, mindful, awake. In recovery, usually used in conjunction
with the word "contact" and refers to a higher power, as in the Eleventh
Step. Varies from person to person and is based on individual experience.
Most often refers to an understanding or feeling that comes from being
mindful of, having faith, or believing that a higher power has one's best
interest in mind and will take care of one's needs. In most twelve-step
programs a conscious (contact) is usually achieved through prayer
and meditation.

CONSISTENT

Constant, steady, dependable. To do something on a regular basis.
The recovery process requires that one meet a few basic requirements
on a consistent basis, such as not using, working the steps, attending
meetings, and calling a sponsor.

CONTRIBUTION

Donation, offering, gift. To provide financially or offer one's time to a
cause or situation. In recovery terms, to give of one's resources (financial
and/or personal as in sponsorship, helping to clean up a room after a
meeting, performing service for the fellowship, etc.). The principle of
contribution is discussed in the Seventh Tradition and referred to as
"self-supporting through our own contributions."

CONTROL

Dominate, have power over, restrain. To attempt to exert power or
influence over or to make decisions for another. In recovery terms,
attempting to control the circumstances or people in one's life is the
opposite of surrender and/or acceptance. Many people, before entering
recovery, believed they had control over their lives and addiction until they
surrendered and accepted their powerlessness as stated in the First Step.

CONTROVERSY

Disagreement, debate, storm. Controversy exists when groups or persons are at odds or there are situations causing strife and contention. Some issues are more controversial than others. Controversy can occur when people have strong feelings or beliefs about a particular topic of discussion. The Tenth Tradition cautions twelve-step members and groups to avoid being drawn into public controversy.

CONVENTION

A meeting, gathering, get-together. A gathering of program members held to celebrate or discuss recovery. Most twelve-step programs usually have some type of convention on a local, state, regional, and/or international/world level. Also referred to as "conference" in Alcoholics Anonymous. A convention can also be a standard, rule, or custom.

COPE

Handle, manage, address. The action of dealing with, addressing, or getting through a difficult situation, whether the situation be illness, financial troubles, relationship issues, death of a loved one, etc.

COUNSELOR

Therapist, advisor, psychoanalyst. A person who has been trained or certified to counsel others in a particular area of concern, e.g., family and marriage issues, substance abuse, mental health disorders, debt, etc. There are no counselors or professionals in twelve-step programs, other than as fellowship members.

COURAGE

Valor, bravery, nerve. The spiritual principle of remaining steadfast and undeterred through adversity or hardship. Attempting to persevere through one's fear in order to accomplish a goal.

CRISIS

Predicament, disaster, catastrophe. An emergency or critical situation. Many people find themselves in crisis because of the damage caused by their active addiction. A crisis can be medical, financial, marital, emotional, physical, etc.

CRITICAL

Judgmental, unsympathetic, fault-finding. Judging self or others severely, reproaching, blaming, or disparaging. This reference is considered a character defect. Also refers to being essential or important.

CROSSTALK

Term used in many twelve-step meetings that refers to speaking out of turn. This may include carrying on a conversation with one's neighbors, "answering" another member who has just shared, or not waiting for a speaker to finish sharing, but interrupting him or her to offer a rebuttal or give advice. Texting may also be considered crosstalk in some meetings, according to the group's conscience. Though meeting formats vary according to each autonomous group's conscience, crosstalk is universally frowned upon and discouraged in twelve-step meetings, as is any other behavior that can distract those who wish to participate from hearing the message of recovery.

CRYSTAL METH ANONYMOUS (CMA)

A twelve-step fellowship of men and women who wish to recover from addiction to crystal meth. The only requirement for membership is a desire to stop using. The CMA recovery text is currently in the process of being written. The working title is *Unspun: Stories of Hope from Crystal Meth Anonymous.*

The first meeting of Crystal Meth Anonymous was held on September 16, 1994 in West Hollywood, California. Currently, there are approximately 500 meetings in the US, Canada, and Australia.

CULT

Usually refers to a religious group or subgroup of a larger religion. A faction or sect. Often isolationist and fervent in nature and prone to worshipping or following a single figurehead and/or object. Sometimes inaccurately used to characterize twelve-step programs. Fellowship members are free to follow their own consciences and equally free to leave at any time. Members are devoted, but membership is never coerced.

CUTTING

Self-mutilation or self-harm carried out in order to relieve emotional stress, pain, or suffering. May not be "cutting" with a blade *per se*, but may take other forms such as "accidents," burnings, scaldings, and other deliberate, direct injuries to one's own body that cause tissue damage and that arise out of an attempt to deal with overwhelmingly distressing situations or past trauma.

May become addictive as the endorphins released as a result of the pain sensation create a "high" and the physical pain momentarily overrides the cutter's/mutilator's emotional pain. No discrete, formal, twelve-step programs exist, but mental health professionals are becoming more aware of this condition.

Dd

DAILY

Every day, once every twenty-four hours, once a day. Members in twelve-step programs practice recovery on a daily basis, one day at a time.

DEATH

The end of life; a cessation of existence in the physical world. Usually spoken of as one of the three likely fates of an addict who continues to use/abuse drugs and does not start recovery, the others being jails or institutions. There is also death of a spiritual nature as the result of using a substance or acting on a particular behavior in active addiction; however, this spirit may be rekindled through the application of the Twelve Steps.

DEBTORS ANONYMOUS (DA)

Debtors Anonymous is a twelve-step fellowship of men and women whose primary purpose is to stop "compulsive debting." Developed by early members of AA who, at that time, were suffering financial consequences that were the result of actions they had taken while drinking. These members sought to focus on becoming financially responsible in recovery. The Twelve Steps of DA convey the same message as other twelve-step fellowships: recovery is possible through adherence to a few simple directions and trust in a higher power.

DECEPTION

Fraud, dishonesty, ruse. To be dishonest in order to conceal certain actions or behaviors one wishes to hide due to feeling shame or guilt. The result of a lack of courage to face the necessary consequences, resulting in more lies (deceptions), which compound upon one another and ultimately may lead to relapse.

DECISION

Conclusion, verdict, choice. To come to some resolution in one's mind that it is time to take a certain action. To choose to do something. In terms of the Third Step, it is referred to as an action rather than a thought.

DEFECT(S)

Imperfection(s), flaw(s), fault(s). Character defects are usually identified while writing the Fourth Step, clarified when sharing that writing with a sponsor in the Fifth Step, and addressed in the Sixth and Seventh Steps. In twelve-step terms, character defects may be negative behaviors from which people in recovery derive immediate gratification while causing pain or destruction to self or others. Defects harm relationships and keep an individual isolated. Isolation gives the disease more control over one's behavior and ultimately can lead a person in a twelve-step program to relapse. Character defects may stand in the way of developing a relationship with a higher power.

DEFENSE/DEFENSIVE

Guard, protection, security. Frequently used in conjunction with the psychological/behavioral term "defense mechanism." This refers to the way in which a person copes with a specific occurrence and/or event. Active addiction often causes these defense mechanisms to be out-of-balance and/or exaggerated.

To be defensive is to be exaggeratedly self-protective, suspicious, distrustful. Constantly protecting oneself from criticism, exposure of one's shortcomings, or other real or perceived threats to the ego. Intended to withstand or deter aggression or attack. Though defensiveness can be a natural, normal response to feeling attacked, it is generally considered a character defect.

DEGRADATION

Disgrace, ruin, humiliation. An unacceptable state or condition of mind and body that usually comes as a result of losing what was formerly esteemed by a person in active addiction. May include material possessions, human relationships, attributes, etc.

DELUSION

False impression, misconception, illusion. A state of mind in which an individual believes that imaginary things are real or vice-versa. Delusions are distorted beliefs. In the extreme, they have no basis in reality and can be a psychotic disorder. Not to be confused with hallucinations; delusions are more like fantasies in which an addict sees him- or herself as either more of a victim or more heroic than he or she actually is.

Addiction is often said to be a disease of perception, and the perceptions of addicts are generally skewed. The humorous expression, "it's all about me," used in the rooms of recovery is really an accurate description of the view of the world from someone in active addiction, which is typically egocentric, childish, and deluded in the extreme.

DEMANDING

Challenging, needy, dissatisfied. Requiring much effort or attention. To ask for urgently or peremptorily. Claiming as one's due. Considered a character defect.

DEMORALIZATION

Deflation, undermining, discouragement. Usually the result of compromising one's morals or principles in order to satisfy an immediate need be it for alcohol or other drugs, gambling, shopping, sex, etc. Engaging in acts out of desperation, which would otherwise disgust an individual under normal circumstances. Most often experienced as a direct result of active addiction. Also refers to a feeling of discouragement or disenfranchisement as related to employment, relationships, etc.

DENIAL

Refutation, rebuttal, disavowal. Denial is a defense mechanism a person uses so that he or she can continue to use addictively. It is, in fact, considered one of the primary presenting symptoms of addiction by many experts. An inability to accept reality and/or truth. Usually not conscious until external circumstances cause an insight or an awakening. A person in denial may be fully aware of a destructive pattern of behavior, but may minimize or underestimate the impact of the pattern on his or her life. Until denial is overcome the individual most often will be unwilling to confront his or her addiction.

DEPENDENCY

Addiction, reliance, habit. Unhealthy need for a behavior or substance, mental, or physical in nature, that results in severe withdrawal that may be physical or psychological and often requires some type of detoxification. Emotional or other attachment to a behavior that provides a false sense of security or that fills a perceived and perhaps distorted need, and is therefore difficult to stop or break free from.

DEPRESSED ANONYMOUS

A twelve-step fellowship that was formed with the idea that mutual aid empowers people and is a therapeutic healing force. Depressed Anonymous offers depressed individuals information on how to work on overcoming depression. It seeks to inform and educate the public about the signs and symptoms of depression, inform them of where they can go to seek help, and provide educational and advocacy resources to professionals so that they may provide their patients with hope and real help.

DEPRAVITY

Decadence, corruption, immorality. To be morally perverted; corrupted; lacking in virtues or principles. Indicative of the circumstances to which active addiction often brings a person.

DEPRESSION

Despair, misery, hopelessness. Feelings of extreme sadness, as in chronic depression, which involves a chemical imbalance in the brain often requiring treatment with medication. Symptoms of depression may be: lethargy, sadness, loss of motivation, loss of appetite, hopelessness, fear, etc. May be chronic or situational. Situational depression usually does not require medication and may be alleviated with the use of any of various forms of psychotherapy; it usually will pass when the situation causing it does.

DERELICTION

Negligence, delinquency, disregard. Refers to neglect of things such as job or family responsibilities, etc. The word "derelict," for "hobo," "tramp," or "bum," means one whose life is in ruins, who is abandoned or has abandoned a productive life, and/or whose basic life needs are neglected or have been destroyed. May be caused by someone living in active addiction.

DESIRE

Longing, yearning, want. A craving for something; to long or hope for. Sometimes viewed in negative terms; however, in twelve-step programs, "desire" is the only requirement for membership, as in "desire to stop using/drinking/gambling/eating compulsively/etc."

DESPAIR

The very pit of hopelessness, despondency, gloom. To feel anguished, lost, confused. Many twelve-step programs consider despair to be caused by lack of a relationship with a higher power. A feeling one has when acting out on character defects and/or not working a program of recovery; the result of a negative or maladaptive behavior.

DESPERATION

Extreme anxiety, worry, abject fear. The feeling of "if I don't get what I need, I will die," either coupled with some type of obsession or compulsion or the result of an obsession or compulsion. Most commonly associated with active addiction and typical of those seeking more of the substance/behavior to which they are addicted. In recovery terms, may also relate to an individual who is desperate to get clean/sober or stop acting on certain behaviors.

DESTRUCTIVE

Damaging, detrimental, injurious. Causing harm or creating ruin. Destructive behavior is a common component of active addiction.

DETACH

Disconnect, disengage, to separate from a person, group, thing, or place. Usually used in reference to removing oneself from something that may be deemed harmful, unhealthy, or dangerous.

DETOX (from DETOXIFY)

To remove or rid the body of poisons, usually in reference to toxic (poisonous) and/or addictive substances, particularly alcohol and/or other drugs Also refers to a medical facility dealing specifically with the removal of alcohol and/or other drugs from the body in a controlled and medically-supervised environment.

DILEMMA

Predicament, tight spot, impasse. In recovery terms, dilemmas may relate to a crisis of conscience as a result of the conflict between old and new ways of life or old and new values and behaviors.

DIRECTION

Path, course, route. Instructions and/or suggestions on how to accomplish a task or arrive at a location. May include the suggestions given to a recovering person to assist him or her with staying in recovery.

DISAGREEMENT

Difference of opinion, dispute, quarrel. Disagreements do not have to be catastrophic. One of the lessons recovery teaches: friends can disagree and remain friendly.

DISAPPOINTMENT

Discontent, frustration, dissatisfaction. Feeling let down or sad about the outcome of a situation. Often occurs when expectations are not met. A feeling that may occur when life happens rather than what one would prefer to have happen.

DISCIPLINE

Order, restraint, punishment. Adherence to a code of beliefs and/ or values. To hold oneself to a standard of actions, principles, etc. In recovery terms, discipline may refer to the consistent performance of certain actions such as praying, meditating, calling one's sponsor, going to recovery meetings, and not using mind- or mood-altering substances or engaging in maladaptive, compulsive behaviors.

DISCONNECT(ED)

To sever or interrupt a link or relationship, for example between self and others or self and one's higher power. To experience a feeling of alienation or isolation.

DISCRETION

Good judgment, prudence, caution. Diplomacy, tact, the ability to make good choices. Discretion also can help an individual decide what to share with others in meetings and what is better shared privately with a sponsor.

DISEASE (OF ADDICTION)

Ailment, sickness, syndrome. The disease concept of the nature of addiction and alcoholism is recognized by the American Medical Association and World Health Organization, putting to rest the old idea that addiction is a mental or moral failing.

In recovery, reference to "the disease" commonly means addiction—the threefold disease affecting body, mind, and spirit. It is chronic, progressive, incurable, and fatal if left untreated. The application of the twelve-step recovery model is considered one of the more successful treatments for the disease of addiction since it addresses the mind, body, and spirit of recovering individuals. Without any type of treatment, addiction is most likely to be fatal.

DISHONESTY

Untruthfulness, deceit, lying. Often regarded as one of the more difficult practices to change for a person in recovery, since dishonesty/lying is one of the characteristics of active addiction. Can also be practiced by commission (lying) or omission (hiding) of the truth. Considered a character defect.

DISHONOR/DISHONORABLE

To destroy another's reputation (to dishonor). Lacking integrity, unprincipled, shameful. Behavior that is unethical.

DISSATISFIED

Malcontent, disgruntled, discontented. Having expectations that never seem to be met, displeased or frustrated. Chronic dissatisfaction is considered a character defect.

DISTURBING

Troubling, alarming, distressing. Something that agitates/disturbs the senses or makes one ill (on a physical, mental, emotional, or spiritual level) or causes discomfort. Causing stress or concern.

DIVERSITY

Assortment, range, mixture. In modern parlance, "diversity" refers to the myriad ethnic, religious, age, gender, economic, educational, and other differences that mark the members of a societal group as distinct from each other. In addiction and in recovery, the entire spectrum of human experience is contained; no group is immune or exempt. Addiction can happen to anyone, and so can recovery.

DIVINE

Of God, God-like, heavenly. Recovery is often referred to as a God-given gift or a gift from a higher power. Also refers to a blessing or miracle believed to come from some otherworldly source not of one's own making or doing.

DOGMA

An explicitly expressed belief, a manifesto, a creed. Often considered rigid and inflexible. A directive to act a certain way because it is believed some supreme being or religious practice demands it. In recovery, certain beliefs are very rigidly held by some groups, as if they are "carved in stone" and subject to only one interpretation. Some people, likewise, may be very rigid in their practice of their particular program of recovery.

DOPE-FIENDING

The action of manipulating a situation and/or person in order to get something. A slang term for doing something that is usually underhanded or unethical, to get one's (addictive) needs met. Behavior seen most readily in those still in active addiction.

DOUBT

Uncertainty, reservation, misgiving. To be undecided about something. Many people who are new to recovery often doubt that a program as simple as twelve-step fellowships can actually help them heal from the disease of addiction.

DRAMATIC

Inauthentic, staged, exaggerated. Overly expressive or emotional; theatrical. Considered a character defect when used excessively.

DREAMS

Aspirations, hopes, images. Also refers to the brain activity that occurs during REM (rapid eye movement) sleep. Something to strive and work toward. Many in recovery speak of "dreams that come true," in reference to those ideas or hopes that were lost in active addiction. Those new to recovery often speak about "using" or "drunk" dreams in which they use alcohol or other drugs or engage in addictive behavior. These "using" dreams can be very realistic in nature and cause distress. "Using" dreams can occasionally happen to anyone in recovery regardless of time in the program and are no more predictive of actual future behavior than any other dream.

DRUGS

Medicinal or medical substances. Also refers to any number of mind- and/or mood-altering chemicals and substances, including alcohol. A habit-forming substance. May be prescribed by a health care provider or obtained illegally.

DRY/DRY DRUNK

To be free from alcohol. Abstinence from alcohol. Also refers to someone in Alcoholics Anonymous who is not actively working the AA program and is miserable and/or unhappy, as in a "dry drunk."

DUAL DIAGNOSIS

Mental illness or intellectual disability existing concurrently with addiction. Numerous theories exist to explain the relationship between co-occurring mental illness and substance abuse, including causality (the theory that certain substances induce mental disorders), multiple risk factors (social isolation, poverty, etc.), self-medication (use of substances to alleviate symptoms of mental disorders), and others. Diagnosis and treatment can be challenging, as substance abuse itself often induces psychiatric symptoms. Twelve-step fellowships do not treat mental health disorders; members in need of counseling are encouraged to seek treatment from a mental health or medical professional in addition to attending meetings and working the steps.

DUAL RECOVERY ANONYMOUS (DRA)

A twelve-step organization for people with a dual diagnosis. There are only two requirements for membership: a desire to stop using alcohol or other intoxicating drugs and a desire to manage emotional or psychiatric illness in a healthy and constructive way. The first DRA meeting was held in Kansas in 1989. The fellowship's recovery text is titled, *The Dual Disorders Recovery Book*.

DYNAMIC(S)

Vibrant, energetic, forceful. Able to change. Various components or sides of a situation in movement together. All the parts of a scenario that make up its value; different qualities, or complexities of a given situation.

Ee

EGO

The self, sometimes thought of as the personality, sense of self, or the "I" of existence. The way one views oneself as in self-image or self-esteem. Can refer to an exaggerated sense of self, an inflated view or opinion of oneself or a destructive and hurtful view of self.

EGOCENTRIC

Self-obsessed, self-centered, self-absorbed. Focused on oneself, not considerate of others. Selfish. Considered a character defect.

EIGHTH STEP

From the Twelve Steps (Step Eight). Practicing this step means listing all those people and institutions one harmed during active addiction and becoming willing to make amends to all of them. These amends may be direct or indirect, and may include financial as well as emotional amends.

EIGHTH TRADITION

From the Twelve Traditions (Tradition Eight). A guideline stating that twelve-step programs should always be nonprofessional, but that their service centers (central offices or service headquarters) are permitted to employ "special workers" to conduct the everyday business of the center. These employees may or may not be program members themselves.

ELEVENTH STEP

From the Twelve Steps (Step Eleven). The primary focus of this step is for the individual to practice regular prayer and meditation in order to seek a "conscious contact" with a higher power so that the individual can have knowledge of a higher power's will and the power/courage to carry out that will.

ELEVENTH TRADITION

From the Twelve Traditions (Tradition Eleven). A guideline for twelve-step programs stating that the programs' public relations policies must be based on members' demonstrated behavior in recovery rather than by active promotion, recruitment, or advertisement of their recovery. Also states that individuals should always maintain their personal anonymity in every medium; however, the decision to break one's anonymity to help another is always left to the individual program member.

EMOTIONAL

Poignant, touching, moving. To be moved by feelings rather than pure reason or intellect; expressive, sensitive, open, demonstrative. To have feelings, be affected by feelings, or to make decisions based on feelings. May imply coming from the heart (feeling) as opposed to from the head (intellect).

EMOTIONS

Sensations, passion; feelings such as sadness, joy, love, pain, fear, happiness, loneliness, guilt, etc. Any number of complex chemical responses stemming from the brain as a reaction to a particular situation, event, thought, etc.

EMOTIONS ANONYMOUS (EA)

Emotions Anonymous is a twelve-step fellowship composed of men and women who come together for the purpose of working toward recovery from emotional difficulties such as depression, anger, broken or strained relationships, grief, anxiety, low self-esteem, panic, debilitating fears, etc. EA was founded in 1971 in St. Paul, Minnesota and currently has approximately 1,000 chapters in thirty-five countries, including the US. The title for the fellowship's recovery text is *Emotions Anonymous*.

EMPATHY/EMPATHIZE

Identification, understanding, compassion/to relate to another as a fellow human. The ability to identify with another; to put oneself in another's position; to "walk in another's shoes." The key to unlocking the twelve-step process, as members listen to and identify with others in the program and gain the hope that what worked for the others will also work in their own lives.

ENABLE

Permit, make possible, allow. To assist in accomplishing a task or maintaining a way of life.

The word *enable* forms the basis for *enabler*, which defines individuals who, often believing they are helping someone with addiction, give that person money, food, shelter, or some other form of assistance. The enabler invariably only helps the person in active addiction to continue to use. Enablers are usually the parents, other family members, close friends, or loved ones of those who are addicted.

ENDORSE

Approve, sanction, support. Financial payment, as in monetary sponsorship. Give a stamp of approval and/or backing to a thing (person, place, institution, political party, etc.). Twelve-step programs do not endorse other programs, facilities, or institutions as cautioned in the Sixth Tradition because of the danger that the message of the twelve-step program may be diluted or misrepresented.

ENVY

Covetousness, desire, resentful longing. A feeling of discontent and resentment aroused by the desire for the possessions or qualities of another. Considered a character defect.

EQUALITY

Impartiality, sameness, parity. Treatment of all people in the same manner. Also refers to equivalence, uniformity, and/or similarity. All members of twelve-step programs are equal, no matter how much time in recovery they may have. There are no "leaders" or "bosses."

ESCAPISM

Distraction, avoidance, diversion. The tendency to get away from reality or routine by indulging in daydreaming, fantasizing, or entertainment. Active addiction provides a form of escapism because it prevents the individual from facing his or her reality. Considered a character defect.

ESOTERIC

Mysterious, cryptic, obscure. Unfamiliar, out-of-the-ordinary. Understood by a select few, e.g., a "secret society." Twelve-step recovery is the opposite of esoteric because there are no secret doctrines or membership requirements other than a desire to stop using. All the tenets and history of twelve-step recovery are open to anyone who wishes to learn about them, and many meetings are open to the public.

ESKIMO

Term used in AA, taken from the Big Book, (the chapter "Working with Others") where an unidentified, fictitious "Eskimo" might turn up in the frozen north with a bottle that might tempt an alcoholic who was not in fit spiritual condition. Confusingly, this word is sometimes used by AA fellowship members to refer to the person who first carried the message of recovery to them or the person who physically saved their lives. This

term can be thought of in a general way as referring to the person who
brings one what is needed, spiritually or physically, or who challenges
one to remain in recovery.

ETHICS

Values, principles, morals. A code to live by, moral standards, a set
of guiding principles based on individual morals or the morals of a
society or community; rightness of conduct either by an individual or
organization. Many professional organizations have governing guidelines
to ensure ethical conduct, such as the American Medical Association,
the American Bar Association, etc. In recovery, the Twelve Steps teach
members to develop healthy standards/ethics by which to live.

EUPHORIC RECALL

Exaggerated and/or distorted positive memories of previous using
experiences during active addiction. Often euphoric recall interferes with
the accurate recollection of the negative consequences of using.

EXACT

Accurate, literal, to be precise and specific. To be clear and
straightforward in description. In relation to a Fifth, Eighth, and Ninth
Step, to be precise and to explain the specific nature of the wrong and
the harm one has done, to whom and why.

EXERCISE

To implement, take action, put into effect. Also refers to working out
(as in physically exercising or training). To perform some physical,
mental, or spiritual action repeatedly in order to build strength, whether
physical, social, mental, or spiritual.

EXPECTATION

Prospect, hope, anticipation. The state of wanting something from a person, event, or thing. The belief that one will derive a certain benefit from a certain action. Hoping to get one's needs met in the way one wants; may cause a desire for unrealistic outcomes.

EXPERIENCE

Know-how, skill, understanding. The knowledge obtained from living through events. The accumulation of everything that has happened in one's past. Past occurrence. The process of actually going through something rather than hearing about it, reading about it, or watching it.

EXTREMISM

Radicalism, fanaticism, fervor. Advocating or resorting to measures beyond the norm. Making situations or conditions appear much more or much less than what they are. As related to recovery, the Twelve Steps teach members to avoid extremism by finding balance in their lives physically, mentally, emotionally, and spiritually. Considered a character defect.

re•cov•er•y |ri'kəvərē|

Ff

FAITH

Conviction, confidence, trust. Belief that is not based on actual evidence/proof. A reliance and/or belief (especially in God or a higher power). The act of having a conscious relationship with a higher power; to believe through experience or trust that the best or highest good will happen in one's life as a result of that relationship.

FAMILIES ANONYMOUS (FA)

Families Anonymous is a twelve-step fellowship for families and friends whose lives have been adversely affected by a loved one's addiction to alcohol or other drugs. The first FA group met in 1971 in California, and today has over 200 groups in the US and 300 international groups in twenty countries. *Today a Better Way* is the fellowship's recovery text.

FAMILY

Ancestors, relatives, kin. A group of people who are connected, whether by blood, circumstance, or choice. Many members in twelve-step fellowships consider fellow members as part of their family.

FAMILY OF ORIGIN WORK

Refers to the process of examining one's childhood in order to heal from the past and move on in recovery. Sometimes, but not necessarily a part of addiction recovery, but often useful for those in recovery whose childhoods included trauma (physical, sexual, or emotional abuse) or a chaotic or neglectful living environment. Typically provided in the context of professional counseling and/or therapy.

FANTASY

Flight of the imagination, unreality, dream. Something not based in reality. A daydream. Fantasies can become problematic in recovery when they interfere with people's ability to live in the moment.

FATIGUE

Lack of energy, exhaustion, weariness. The state of being extremely tired or run down. Can be experienced on an emotional, spiritual, mental, and/or physical level. May stem from any number of physiological and/or psychological causes such as poor eating habits, lack of proper rest or sleep, stress (physical/emotional/mental/spiritual), active addiction, withdrawal, etc.

FAULTS

Errors, wrongs, flaws. One's faults are not one's past actions; they are another name for the character defects that are the root causes of one's actions. They are the negative qualities, such as greed, lust, or pride, which led to the actions that hurt others and oneself. The fault of "greed," for example, may have led one to theft, or the fault of "lust" may have led one to cheat on a partner.

There is no one on earth without faults; our faults, some say, are what make us human. Sometimes our faults can lead us, through suffering, to do good or to benefit others by our experiences; so no one need feel ashamed of discovering faults in themselves. The only shameful thing is to know one has faults and do nothing about them.

FEAR

Anxiety, terror, dread. The quality or state of being frightened, anxious, or scared. Fear can be of future events, outcomes (real or imagined) based on past harms, or projection of future harms. Fear is at the root of many other emotions and character defects.

In recovery, the word fear is often used as an acronym, "**F**orget **E**verything **A**nd **R**un," to describe the attitude toward life's difficulties that persons in recovery may have taken in active addiction. A person in recovery may feel fear, but uses the tools of the program to confront the life events that he or she would formerly have run from in fear. The positive form of this acronym is "**F**ace **E**verything **A**nd **R**ecover."

FEARLESS

The state of being bold, daring, without anxiety or nervousness. The proper approach to one's Fourth Step inventory is to be "searching and fearless" when looking over past wrongs. In order to grow in recovery, one should not shrink from looking at his or her past actions, no matter how painful it is to do so; one must be fearless in looking at the truth about him- or herself to reap the greatest benefit from a Fourth Step.

FEELINGS

Emotions, sentiments, sensations. Common examples include happiness, sadness, pride, embarrassment, bliss, joy, elation, gratitude, etc. Persons in recovery may not be used to actually *feeling* their emotions, having masked them with the substances or activities to which they were addicted. Avoidance of feelings is one reason many people give when asked why they began using in the first place.

Feelings may be overwhelming in early recovery as they begin to resurface, and even positive feelings should be shared, with a sponsor, in a meeting, or with a counselor or other support-system member. Feelings are nothing to fear, although it may feel as if they are when they first emerge.

FEES

Charges, payments, costs. Money given in exchange for membership in a group or organization or a sum paid to obtain goods or services. Twelve-step fellowships do not charge any fees for membership according to their own traditions. Any donations members give at meetings are voluntary and are given to enable the groups to support themselves.

FELLOWSHIP/FELLOWSHIPPING

Camaraderie, association, comradeship. A voluntary association of people joined together by a common desire, problem, interests, wants, needs, circumstances, etc.

Fellowshipping in twelve-step terms refers to the act of gathering with other people in a twelve-step program for social activities such as eating, going out for coffee, or for fun and recreation. Spending time with people in one's twelve-step program outside of a meeting setting.

FIFTH STEP

From the Twelve Steps (Step Five). Requires persons in recovery to admit—to their higher power, to another person (usually a sponsor), and to themselves—the exact nature of their wrongs. During this step, the person in recovery traditionally reads or discloses what was written in his or her Fourth Step to a sponsor, but another trusted advisor, such as a clergyperson, may hear the Fifth Step.

FIFTH TRADITION

From the Twelve Traditions (Tradition Five). A guideline for twelve-step programs stating that each group or meeting has one primary purpose, which is to carry the message of the Twelve Steps to the person who still suffers from addiction in any of its manifestations (this may not be a person still in active addiction or even a newcomer—persons in long-term recovery may still suffer and may need the help of another program member).

FIRST STEP

From the Twelve Steps (Step One). This calls for the admission (acknowledgement) that a person seeking recovery is powerless over his or her addiction (or manifestation of addiction) and that his or her life has become unmanageable. Said to be the only step that must be "worked perfectly." It is the basis and foundation for recovery, as the logical action flowing from admitting powerlessness over one's addiction is to abstain from the substance or behavior to which he or she is addicted. Only when one abstains can recovery begin to work in one's life. Only when a person admits to his or her "innermost self" that he or she is powerless can recovery begin.

FIRST TRADITION

From the Twelve Traditions (Tradition One). A guideline for twelve-step programs that states that the common welfare of the program should come first and that the recovery of the individual depends on the strength, stability, and unity of the twelve-step program. This is based on the belief that the program or fellowship must live or its members will not. Therefore, the traditions were developed and adopted to ensure that what worked for the program's founders will be carried on to future generations without being changed or interfered with simply for the sake of change.

FLASHBACK

Intermittent, unsought and usually unwelcome memories of past experiences that can happen even after years in recovery. May be more common for those who have used hallucinogenic drugs. These can be frightening, but do not indicate that a person is about to experience a relapse. Like any other unusual feeling, a flashback should probably be discussed with a sponsor. If frequency and intensity is interrupting one's daily functions, a discussion with a medical professional to ensure there is no underlying physical or mental illness might be a consideration.

In psychology, a flashback can be a symptom of Post-Traumatic Stress Disorder.

FLEXIBLE

Elastic, supple, lithe. Having the ability to bend, compromise, or adjust to a changing situation. Also refers to a mental state that allows a person to approach the recovery journey with the open-mindedness and willingness required to succeed.

FOOD ADDICTS ANONYMOUS (FAA)

A twelve-step organization that believes food addiction is a biochemical disorder that cannot be cured by willpower or therapy alone. Members believe that food addiction can be managed by abstaining from (eliminating) addictive foods, following a program of healthy nutrition, and working the Twelve Steps of the program. FAA's members' primary purpose is to stay abstinent and help other food addicts to achieve abstinence. There is a recovery text called The Green Book that describes the FAA program and plan for recovery.

FOOTWORK

Preparations, groundwork, skillful foot action. The necessary work and actions associated with what one must do in order to work and stay in a program of recovery. Usually said in reference to going to meetings, getting a sponsor, and working steps. Might also refer to living life on life's terms, preparing to find a job by getting training, sticking to a budget to save money for things one wants, etc.

Many in recovery say, "I'm in the footwork business; my higher power is in the results business," to indicate their acknowledgement that even though they are responsible for doing the footwork of recovery (or of living), they are powerless over the results and must leave those up to their higher power.

FORGIVE/FORGIVENESS

Absolve, pardon, excuse. To relinquish resentments or grudges one has for another person, group, society, or concept.

Forgiveness is the act of or intention to be forgiving and can be extended to others whether or not they apologize or make amends. To hold onto resentments or grudges without forgiveness hurts only the one who holds them; therefore, practicing forgiveness is an important part of the healing process for most people in recovery. Step Eight and Step Nine discuss the importance of forgiveness in one's recovery program.

FOUNDATION

Groundwork, base, underpinning. Firm footing on which to build a recovery program; establishing a connection with a regular meeting or group and with friends and peers in recovery, taking a service position, getting a sponsor, and working steps. Attending "ninety meetings in ninety days" is a time-tested formula recommended to newcomers wishing to establish a firm foundation in recovery.

FOURTH STEP

From the Twelve Steps (Step Four). Calls for a "searching and fearless" moral inventory. The particulars of working this step may vary according to fellowship attended. For example, some fellowships have members write a narrative/biography or make a list, or write in side-by-side columns, but whatever format is followed, the Fourth Step inventory is a written assessment by a person in recovery of his or her own past deeds, revealing resentments, strengths and weaknesses, character defects, and all aspects of his or her relationships, as well as character assets. The point is to examine one's character and to get rid of what is damaged and determine what needs to be built up for continued healthy growth.

The Fourth Step is often approached with great fear by the newcomer, but there is no need for this. All the millions of people, all over the world, who have achieved lasting, long-term recovery through twelve-step programs, have taken Fourth Steps. While writing down one's past deeds might be embarrassing or even emotionally upsetting, it is never going to be as bad as having done those deeds in the first place. As old timers say, "If there's a word for what you've done, then you're not the first or the only person to have done it." An understanding sponsor will be of great help in taking this step.

Old timers, some of whom have gone through the steps, including the Fourth Step, numerous times, insist that the Fourth Step is where true relief from the suffering of addiction begins.

FOURTH TRADITION

From the Twelve Traditions (Tradition Four). A guideline for twelve-step programs stating that each group and meeting should be self-regulating, except regarding issues that affect other groups, meetings, or the twelve-step program itself. Groups hold regular business meetings to autonomously determine the rules and format for their particular group's meetings and take votes, called "group consciences," to settle any issues. These only apply to the particular group itself; not to the program as a whole.

FOXHOLE PRAYERS

Adapted from the old saying, "there are no atheists in foxholes." The idea behind the saying is that a soldier in a foxhole (a desperate situation) will usually utter a prayer when enemy fire is getting close, even if he or she is not ordinarily prayerful.

A foxhole prayer is the sort of prayer people in active addiction utter in desperation after they are already in a bad situation (usually the result of behavior in active addiction such as incarceration, extreme illness, hospitalization, etc.).

FREEDOM

Independence, liberty, autonomy. The result of living a life based in spiritual principles, working the Twelve Steps, and not being bound by active addiction. Those in recovery live lives that are truly free, guided by the Twelve Steps and the principles of recovery, because they are no longer in bondage to their addiction or to the demands of "self."

FRIEND

Companion, comrade, ally. A person who provides love, support, companionship, or camaraderie. The friendships one makes in recovery are different in quality from the friendships one may have had while in active addiction. Often a person in recovery finds that the people he or she thought were friends have all vanished now that he or she no longer uses. Recovery friendships are based on a shared experience and common purpose, and encompass love, caring, and concern for one another's well-being.

FRIENDSHIP

Camaraderie, companionship, affinity. The relationship between two or more persons based on healthy love, trust, companionship, and camaraderie. A strong bond between people who spend time with each other, communicating with and helping each other, and enjoying each other's company.

FUNDRAISING

Collecting and gathering money for a particular purpose. Many activities in twelve-step programs, such as dances, picnics, yard sales, bazaars, etc., are designed to raise money to support ancillary activities such as printing meeting directories, supporting helplines, or buying recovery literature to distribute to hospitals and institutions.

There are no dues or fees for program membership itself; monies donated at meetings during the observation of the Seventh Tradition go to pay rent for the meeting space, purchase literature for the meeting, purchase whatever refreshments the meeting offers, and any remainder being held as a "prudent reserve" or donated to the fellowship's area or regional service committee to support the ongoing work of the fellowship.

Gg

GAM-ANON

A twelve-step support fellowship for family and friends of compulsive gamblers.

GAMBLERS ANONYMOUS (GA)

A twelve-step fellowship whose primary focus is to help people stop gambling and to help other compulsive gamblers do the same. They only requirement for membership is a desire to stop gambling. Its members believe that gamblers of their type have a progressive illness that if left untreated, will only get worse and lead to prison, insanity, or death.

The first group meeting of Gamblers Anonymous was held on Friday, September 13, 1957, in Los Angeles, California. Since that time, the fellowship has continued to grow and groups can now be found throughout the world. Though the fellowship does not have a primary recovery text, there are several pieces of literature available. To help an individual determine if he or she is a compulsive gambler, a series of questions, known simply as "20 Questions" is offered. Most compulsive gamblers will answer yes to a minimum of seven of these twenty questions.

GIFTS

Presents, donations, offerings given without the expectation of anything in return. Something bestowed on another with the intention of bringing joy, comfort, or uplift. May be material or spiritual and may include attributes or talents, as in "a gift for music."

"The gifts of the program can take us out of the program," is a popular recovery saying indicating that life in recovery can become so good that one may become "too busy," or feel "too cured" to attend meetings, meet service commitments, write, or otherwise work the steps, etc. These omissions are all indicators that a person is most likely on the road to relapse. One must always remember that unless recovery comes first, the "gifts of recovery" will not last.

GLUTTONY

Excessive eating or drinking, voraciousness, over gorging. Considered one of the seven deadly sins according to Judeo-Christian traditions. Considered a character defect.

GOD

Divinity, supernatural being, deity. An all-knowing, ever-present supreme, supernatural entity/being. For many in recovery, their higher power may represent a return to the God of their childhood, or the word "God" may be a kind of useful shorthand for their higher power, easily understood by others to mean an all-powerful source of strength, comfort, inspiration, etc.

In twelve-step programs/meetings, the word God is often used to describe a higher power that is loving, caring, and only wants the best and highest good for the individual.

For some who have difficulty with the traditional concept of God, the word may be thought of as an acronym for **G**ood **O**rderly **D**irection, which is what the twelve-step program provides. A belief in God is not necessary for twelve-step recovery to work; although the steps do encourage one to find a power greater than oneself.

GOD-AWARENESS

Awareness is consciousness, cognizance, or mindfulness. God-awareness is consciousness of a power greater than oneself. One awakens to this "higher power" when one realizes that recovery, which was once so elusive, is now a reality. The power that brought one to recovery is greater than, and outside of, oneself. This awareness or consciousness is developed and strengthened in recovery by the practice of the Twelve Steps, particularly Step Two and Step Eleven.

GOD BOX or GOD BAG

A box or bag that a recovering person may use in order to pair a physical action with a spiritual one. The recovering person might write down on a piece of paper areas of concern, worrying issues, problems, etc. The person places the slip of paper into the box or bag to symbolize the "turning over" of the issue to a higher power. Placing items into the God box or God bag can be compared to saying a prayer.

GOD SHOT

An inexplicable, unusual, and encouraging happening (some might say a coincidence) that indicates to a person in recovery that he or she is being guided by a higher power. Something said to happen by the divine intervention or act of a benevolent being or cosmic conspiracy. Similar to, and used in the same way as, "miracle." Something that in the ordinary course of life does not usually happen.

GOD'S WILL

Will means resolve, determination, or intent. In twelve-step recovery, the recognition that following one's own will has led one to a life of unmanageability and pain is followed by the decision to follow the will of the higher power in the future, as best it can be ascertained.

Philosophers and theologians have spent centuries trying to discern and explain God's will, to no avail; however, many people in and out of recovery agree that actions that accord with God's will are those that are loving, benevolent, helpful, and constructive.

GOODWILL

Benevolence, kindness, care. Wanting and working for what is best for all involved, whether that means a person, group, community, or society. An inherent benefit of working the Twelve Steps and of twelve-step programs is the development of goodwill toward others and the growing ability to experience the goodwill of others when it is directed toward oneself.

GOSSIP

Hearsay, rumors, scandal. Talking (or writing) about others in a negative manner, usually not in their presence; saying things one would not say about a person were the person present. Gossip may include sharing private information about others to cast them in a bad light (betraying trust) or spreading negative information, whether true or false, to gain some benefit for oneself. Sharing intimate details or secrets about others. Engaging in gossip is considered a character defect.

GRACE

A blessing or piece of good fortune, mercy, pardon. In twelve-step recovery, grace usually refers to unearned blessings bestowed by a higher power on those working the program. A gift from a higher power. Twelve-step members will sometimes describe their gratitude for receiving the gift of recovery with the saying, "There, but for the grace of God, go I," in reference to someone still in active addiction.

Grace also can mean physical elegance of movement, refinement, and poise, as opposed to awkwardness, embarrassment, and unease. Persons in recovery often speak of how the program has taught them to walk through life's problems with "grace and dignity."

GRANDIOSITY

Pretentiousness, lavishness, ostentation. Characterized by greatness of scope or intent, or by feigned or affected grandeur. Thinking of oneself and one's accomplishments in an inflated manner, as in "better than others"; pompousness. Considered a character defect.

GRANDSTANDING

Showing off, showboating, "hamming it up." To perform ostentatiously so as to impress an audience. Some members in recovery will "grandstand" during a share in an effort to impress others. Considered a character defect.

GRATEFUL

Appreciative, thankful, indebted. Gratitude, or developing "an attitude of gratitude," is one of the most important tools in the twelve-step recovery toolbox. Since most people with addiction share a common feeling that "more is never enough," developing an attitude of gratitude represents a shift in the thought patterns of a person in recovery. Changing one's thoughts from "is that all there is?" one can begin to approach life with a deep appreciation for the "little things" that was never there before.

Without gratitude for all that life offers, including both the things one perceives as desirable *and* as undesirable, one is apt to become discouraged by the everyday challenges of life, and therefore vulnerable to the compulsion to use again. With an attitude of gratitude, life's problems can be seen for what they are—opportunities for growth. An attitude of gratitude can make the difference between being a cynical, disconnected attendee at twelve-step meetings or being a joyful, connected member of the recovery community.

GRATITUDE

Appreciation, thankfulness, gratefulness. The feeling one has in recovery upon realizing the difference between where one could be in life and where one actually is.

Gratitude can be cultivated by noticing opportunities to appreciate the "little things" that one formerly took for granted or may even have regarded as annoyances. Writing a "gratitude list" every evening before one's daily inventory (Tenth Step) has helped many in recovery realize exactly how much they have to feel grateful for and the benefits of maintaining this important attitude.

GREED

Avarice, insatiable or self-indulgent gluttony, ravenousness. An excessive desire to acquire or possess more than what one needs, especially with respect to material wealth. Considered a character defect.

GRIEF

Anguish, heartache, misery. Extreme sorrow or sadness caused by the loss of something, such as a dream or physical ability or someone important, as in the loss of a parent, loved one, or pet due to death, physical separation, divorce, etc. In early recovery, one may actually feel grief for the loss of the substance or activity to which one was addicted. It may be necessary to discuss this feeling with a sponsor, write/journal about it, or even, as some in recovery have done, write a "goodbye letter" to the substance or activity for which one is grieving.

GROUP(S)

Set, collection, assembly. In recovery terms, refers to a gathering of people who regularly attend scheduled recovery meetings for the purpose of staying free from active addiction and helping others recover. Groups hold meetings at regularly scheduled times and locations; groups form the "fellowship" of twelve-step recovery. The single group a recovering person attends most frequently and for which he or she performs service work is usually considered that person's "home group"; there may be an enrollment sheet/book/list where home group members list their first names, contact numbers, and their length of time in recovery in order to be of help to newcomers.

Attendance at group meetings is the most well-known part of twelve-step recovery, but it is by no means the entirety of recovery; in addition, there is sponsorship, service work, reading approved literature, and of course, step work, including writing and journaling. The group is where a person in recovery finds "experience, strength, and hope," as well as friendship with like-minded persons who share a common interest and goal: to stay in recovery.

Groups exist for all manifestations of addiction, for example Narcotics Anonymous, Alcoholics Anonymous, Overeaters Anonymous, Nicotine Anonymous, Sex-and-Love Addicts Anonymous, and Debtors Anonymous, to name just a few of the more well-known fellowships. There are also fellowships and groups for families and friends of persons in recovery, such as Nar-Anon, Al-Anon, or Gam-Anon.

GROUP CONSCIENCE

The collective belief or decision of a group. It is not just a "group opinion" or majority vote, where the "loudest" voice can often sway others; the opinion of every member is sought, and all opinions are heard before a decision is made. Group conscience is a powerful spiritual concept; it makes it possible for people of diverse backgrounds and experiences to unite in furtherance of their common purpose: to remain in recovery and extend help to those who still suffer and seek recovery. This terminology commonly relates to the service structure found in most twelve-step fellowships.

GROUP SERVICE REPRESENTATIVE (GSR)

A person elected to present the group's business at area service meetings and carry back news from the service meetings to the group; this can refer to upcoming events, changes in meeting places or regulations, service opportunities, and so forth. The GSR is the link between the group and other service bodies of the twelve-step program. This is terminology specific to the service structure found in most twelve-step fellowships.

GROUP STARTER KIT

This kit contains all the literature and other items that a group needs start a new twelve-step meeting. Most area service committees will have some of these kits available to new groups that request them.

GUIDELINES

Strategies, guiding principles, rules. A set of directives, policies, by-laws, etc. These can be verbal, such as guidelines suggested by others who have experience, or written, such as the Twelve Traditions or Twelve Concepts, which can be found in most twelve-step fellowships.

GUILT

Culpability, responsibility, blame. The feeling of remorse for an action, behavior, choice, or way of life. Guilt, if not addressed in step work, can lead to paralyzing feelings of shame that may set the stage for relapse.

re·cov·er·y |ri'kəvərē|

Hh

H&I (HOSPITALS & INSTITUTIONS)

H&I subcommittees are made up of experienced recovering people who take meetings/presentations/panels into facilities where inmates or residents are not able to attend regular meetings. This is terminology specific to the service structure found in most twelve-step fellowships.

HABIT

Routine, custom, pattern. A physical or psychological activity repeated often enough that it occurs without conscious thought. In active addiction, it is the need for or dependence on a substance or activity. There are positive and negative habits; positive habits, such as regular meeting attendance or prayer and meditation, are often referred to as "disciplines."

HALF-MEASURES

Inadequate or ineffective actions, lukewarm or unenthusiastic attempts. Usually described as putting only half of the necessary required effort into what needs to be accomplished, particularly in recovery. Most persons in recovery say they must put at least as much effort into recovery as they did into using. That means full participation in the program—meeting attendance, step work, sponsorship, writing and/or journaling, and service work.

HALFWAY HOUSE

A transitional living situation between a protected environment, such as a residential treatment center, and living fully and freely in society; may be a house, apartment, or other building where people can live with others in recovery while they adjust to life outside a controlled environment. May be coed or single-gender, independently run or affiliated with a church, treatment center, or other organization. Also called "recovery houses," "sober-living houses," or "transitional houses."

HALT(S)

An acronym for the words **H**ungry, **A**ngry, **L**onely, and **T**ired; these physical and mental states often contribute to the desire to pick up. "S" is added for **S**erious to remind people in recovery to take their *program* seriously, but not to take *themselves* that way. The acronym is then HALTS.

HAPPINESS

Joy, delight, gladness. One of the goals of recovery is to live life, "happy, joyous, and free." It is often remarked that if there were any happiness left "out there," the people who are currently in recovery would still be using. However, persons in recovery know that active addiction only ever brings misery; never happiness. True happiness, joy, and freedom are found in recovery, in living a life free of the "bondage of self," in service to others, working the steps of the program of recovery, enjoying life to the fullest without the mask of addiction to stand in the way of life's simple pleasures, living with an "attitude of gratitude," and meeting one's responsibilities with confidence.

HARM

Damage, injure, wound. To hurt a person, group, community, society, organization, etc. with a behavior or action that is wrong or that causes damage—emotional, physical, or mental. In Step Eight, a list is made of "all persons we had harmed." In addiction, it is common to think "I only harmed myself," but in recovery, one realizes that many in one's life were harmed. Step Nine provides the tools to repair these harms and requires that one do so, if doing so will cause no further harm to themselves or others.

HATRED

Loathing, revulsion, detestation. Demonstration of disgust or extreme animosity or hostility. Considered a character defect.

HEAL

Restore to health, cure, repair. Settling differences, reconciling, rebuilding (especially relationships). Healing is one of the goals of recovery. The Twelve Steps offer a path to healing.

HELP

Aid, assistance, support. Twelve-step programs offer help in the form of fellowship, with the experience, strength, and hope of the group providing support and assistance to all those who seek it. Help is always available from one's higher power, if it is sought.

HELPLESSNESS

Vulnerability, weakness, incapacity. Without the necessary means, strength, or ability to take care of oneself. Helplessness is often confused with powerlessness; however, in twelve-step recovery, the distinction is made clear. One is not helpless over one's choices, one is not helpless over one's actions. One is *powerless* over substances and activities of addiction, over others, and over results. For those in recovery, this is a subtle, but important distinction.

HELPLINE/PHONELINE

A telephone service that provides information about area/region twelve-step programs, such as meeting times and locations, to anyone who calls. This is terminology typically refers to the service structure found in most twelve-step fellowships.

HIGHER POWER

A power greater than oneself; a God of one's own understanding. A key concept in twelve-step recovery that may or may not have anything to do with God (a supreme being/entity) or organized religion.

HITTING BOTTOM

Reaching a point in the downward progression of the disease of addiction at which even the person who suffers from addiction realizes he or she has a serious problem. Varies from person to person; may be physical, emotional, material, or social. Considered the point at which active addiction ends, usually when the person has experienced enough pain, degradation, suffering, or consequences that he or she can no longer continue to use.

HOME GROUP

A meeting or group where members in recovery feel most at "home." Almost any twelve-step meeting can be a home group if someone wishes to join as a member. Home group usually refers to the group or meeting that members attend most regularly; the meeting in which members discuss/vote on group, area, regional motions; help run the meeting; celebrate anniversaries/milestones; and accept service commitments. This is terminology specific to the service structure found in most twelve-step fellowships.

HONESTY

Truthfulness, integrity, sincerity. A spiritual principle that calls for truth-telling. It is possible to lie overtly (a lie of commission) or covertly, by withholding the truth (omission). Twelve-step programs call for honesty as part of working a recovery-oriented program. Members in recovery should strive to practice honesty with their sponsor, and, more importantly, with themselves.

HOPE

Anticipation, expectancy, longing. The message of all twelve-step recovery is a message of hope and that there is a solution. Hope is the belief that no matter how bad matters seem at present, there is a way for one's situation to improve; that all is not lost.

HOPELESSNESS

Desperation, bleakness, misery. To be without expectation of improvement. A particularly dangerous emotional state for those in recovery as it may lead to depression and unwillingness to participate in one's own recovery. Hopelessness can be combated by working the Twelve Steps, working with others in recovery, and being of service.

HORROR

Terror, repulsion, disgust. Considering one's past actions in active addiction may cause feelings of horror; working the steps and making amends for past wrongs is a way to overcome these feelings.

HOSTAGE

Prisoner, captive, detainee. Persons in recovery, when sharing, may refer to their partners and others as having been "hostages," so called because their well-being was subject to the feelings, needs, and actions of the addict in active addiction. Even in recovery, it is possible to "take hostages," when one embarks on or focuses on a relationship, hoping for a "fix," instead of working a program of recovery, including working the steps, being of service, and working with a sponsor.

HOW

An acronym for the way in which twelve-step programs work that includes the spiritual principles considered most essential to recovery: Honesty, Open-mindedness, and Willingness.

HUG

Embrace, enfold, hold close. Wrapping one's arms around another person, in greeting, farewell, or as a show of affection. It is a common practice at many twelve-step meetings to hug other members, although there are also a number of fellowships where members simply shake hands. These types of hugs are not intended to be sexual in nature.

HUMBLE/HUMBLY

Unassuming, modest, self-effacing. The state of receptive self-awareness
called for and promoted by the Twelve Steps; the attitude that promotes
gratitude and receptivity to communication with a higher power.
Discussed in the Seventh Step where members "humbly" ask their higher
power to remove their shortcomings.

HUMILITY

Unassuming nature, modesty, humbleness. Accepting both one's own
assets and liabilities. A realistic view of oneself. Displaying grace and
dignity without arrogance or conceit. Considered a spiritual principle.

HURT

Injure, damage, wound. As a description, to be injured, in pain, or
harmed; to feel pain. In active addiction, one has hurt many others as
well as oneself. In recovery, one strives not to hurt others or oneself by
words or actions.

re·cov·er·y |riˈkəvərē|

Ii

IDENTIFICATION/IDENTIFY

Recognition, classification, in twelve-step terms, to empathize.

In twelve-step recovery, to feel connected with another person, group, community, or society through seeing the similarities between them and oneself. The ability to understand, feel the same as, agree with, empathize or sympathize with another person, despite outward differences.

ILLNESS

Poor health, sickness, disease. Addiction is a disease that affects the mind, body, and spirit. It centers in the brain, and affects every part of the physical, emotional, mental, and spiritual well-being of the person in active addiction.

ILLUSION

False impression, fantasy, daydream. Something imaginary appearing to be real, usually created in one's mind to support a fantasy or as the result of inaccurate perception of a situation. Addiction is the disease that tells the sufferer he or she doesn't have it; this illusion is referred to as denial.

IMMATURITY

Infantile behavior, childishness, irresponsibility. The inability to handle situations with emotional, mental, or spiritual balance. Selfishness is one of the hallmarks of immaturity; the inability to delay gratification or think of others rather than solely of one's own feelings, needs, or desires. It is also one of the hallmarks of active addiction.

IMPERATIVE

Vital, crucial, very important. Certain actions are imperative in order for recovery to occur, such as abstinence, working the steps (preferably with a sponsor), going to meetings, sharing honestly with a sponsor, and carrying the message of recovery to others.

IMPERFECTION

Defect, flaw, shortcoming. Imperfections make one human; striving to overcome them is what recovery is all about. Individuals in recovery examine their imperfections or shortcomings in the Sixth and Seventh Steps seeking to have them removed by a higher power.

IMPROVE

To make better, to increase in quality. The Eleventh Step calls for improving one's conscious contact with one's higher power through prayer and meditation.

INCONSIDERATE

Thoughtless, uncharitable, insensitive to the feelings of others. Displaying a lack of care or concern, especially toward others. Considered a character defect.

INCONSISTENCY

Irregularity, contradiction, erratic. Displaying or marked by a lack of regularity. Lacking in correct logical relation; not in agreement or harmony. Considered a character defect.

INCURABLE

Not curable, unchangeable, chronic. Something for which there is no known cure. Addiction is incurable; it can be arrested through the process of recovery, but one is never fully cured. Recovery is a state that must be maintained through the twelve-step process.

INDEPENDENCE

Autonomy, self-rule, freedom. To be on one's own, acting on one's own behalf. The state of being free from external influence or control or not being dependent on a substance or behavior.

INDIRECT

Roundabout, implied, veiled. Implicit in the Ninth Step; when making *direct* amends may cause additional harm to the injured party or to others, or when the injured party is no longer living or is otherwise unavailable, then *indirect* amends are called for. This is a way of making the wrong right that doesn't directly involve the injured party. If one stole from an orphanage that no longer exists, for example, a way to make amends indirectly might be to support a children's charity. Indirect amends may also include living a full and useful life in recovery.

INFERIOR

Lower, lesser, substandard. Describes a feeling, whether perceived or imagined, of being "less than" another person or group. To feel oneself lacking in a quality or qualities, whether physically, mentally, emotionally, or spiritually. A perception of low worth or value.

INFORMATION PAMPHLET (IP)

Short pieces of writing (brochures) that are specifically focused on topics related to recovery; usually available at twelve-step meetings or central/administrative offices and treatment centers for free or for a nominal cost. Topics may include questions to determine whether or not one's use of a substance or activity is indeed addiction, or may speak specifically to a population, such as youth, women, professionals, or gay and lesbian members of the community.

INJURE

Harm, damage, hurt. To hurt a person, group, community, society, organization, etc. with a behavior or action that is wrong or causes damage; emotional, physical, or mental.

INNER CHILD

Concept in psychology that refers to the belief that regardless of age, every person contains within him- or herself the younger version of him- of herself. This "inner child" may be frightened or insecure, and may never have had his or her emotional needs met at the appropriate time. Inner-child work calls for recognizing, listening to, and nurturing this part of the self in order to develop a personality that is fully integrated and mature in recovery.

INNER-CIRCLE BEHAVIORS

In sex and love addiction recovery, "inner circle behaviors" are behaviors that lead to "self-destructive action" and impede spiritual growth for the addict. These behaviors differ from person to person in recovery, are worked out with guidance from a sponsor—they are the behaviors that constitute a "relapse." They may include masturbation, viewing pornography, extra-marital relationships, anonymous sex, or others, if such behaviors impede recovery or cause harm.

INSANITY

Mental illness or incapacity, senselessness, madness. The often irrational actions individuals participate in during active addiction are commonly considered a state of insanity; accompanied by behaviors and attitudes of extreme mental distortion. The Second Step states that an individual in recovery can be "restored to sanity" by embracing the concept of a power greater than him- or herself.

INSECURITY

Self-doubt, uncertainty, lack of confidence. Feeling doubtful, inadequate, or unprotected. Lacking emotional stability or self-confidence; plagued by anxiety. When insecurity prevents someone in recovery from taking healthy risks to change him- or herself, it is then considered a character defect.

INSENSITIVE
Unfeeling, unsympathetic, tactless. Not physically or emotionally sensitive to the needs of others. Emotionally or physically numb. Lacking in sensitivity to the feelings or circumstances of others. Considered a character defect.

INSIDIOUS
Subtle, covertly sinister, gradual and harmful, as is the disease of addiction. Capable of causing death or extreme destruction to oneself or others while seeming benign. Addiction is often referred to as an insidious disease.

INSIGHT
Perception, intuition, acuity. Seeing what is hidden. The ability to see clearly into the nature of a complex person, situation, or idea. Able to see beneath the surface. An addict can gain insight through attending meetings and incorporating the steps into his or her life.

INSOMNIA
Sleeplessness, restlessness, wakefulness. The inability to sleep; often experienced with the withdrawal of chemicals during the beginning days of an addicted person's recovery. This form of insomnia usually passes as the substances are removed from the body. May be related to or associated with emotional distress.

INTANGIBLE
Vague, insubstantial, elusive. Indefinable or indescribable. Beyond reach. Something without a strong physical existence. An "intangible" is often associated with the benefits of recovery, because the life of the spirit is intangible, yet working a program of recovery is all about "building" this intangible and yet vital element of existence.

INTEGRITY

Truth, honor, reliability. Self-honesty, an ethical standard to live by. Doing the right thing for the right reason. From the idea of being "integrated," whole, having matching "insides" and "outsides," which means behaving and acting the same way in different situations (e.g., "behind closed doors"), regardless of the parties involved. Not participating in a behavior one would then be ashamed of revealing to others. Practicing the principles of the Twelve Steps in all one's affairs. Considered a spiritual principle.

INTERDEPENDENCE

Mutual assistance, cooperation, connection. A state of mutual and reciprocal reliance between entities. Characteristic of the sponsor-sponsee relationship, in which each depends upon the other for support and ongoing recovery.

INTERGROUP

"Intergroup" service, as the name implies, involves representatives from various twelve-step groups within a geographic area meeting together to exchange information and get reports about current events and concerns in other twelve-step groups within their fellowship, locally, nationally, or internationally. Monetary donations are made at such meetings from the group treasuries to help fund services at a state, national, and international level. All who wish to attend are usually welcome to observe, but only elected fellowship members are permitted to vote. This is terminology specific to the service structure found in many twelve-step fellowships.

INTERNET ADDICTION

Internet addiction (also referred to as Internet Dependency or Internet Compulsivity) is an online-related, compulsive behavior that interferes with normal living and causes severe negative consequences in one or more areas of the addict's life.

Most at risk are those who suffer from other manifestations of addiction, such as using alcohol and/or other drugs, smoking, sex, etc. Depression and anxiety-related disorders are also risk factors.

Cybersex, cyberporn, and online affairs are some forms that Internet addiction can take. Gambling and role-playing games, anonymous "chat" rooms, and online shopping may be other manifestations, although more are sure to come to light as humans find more ways to use the Internet. Research is ongoing and practitioners are becoming more aware of the issue. At the time of this writing, there are no specific twelve-step fellowships for Internet addiction, although at one point there was one called Webaholics Anonymous.

INTERVENTION

Intercession, involvement, coming between. The formal process of "coming between" a person in active addiction and his or her addiction. A confrontation between the person with addiction and individuals affected by his or her addiction, often mediated by trained professionals with expertise in conducting and directing these interventions; they are called "interventionists."

INTIMACY

Familiarity, closeness, understanding. Something of a personal or private nature, something that is familiar. Sharing personal information with another person. Intimacy often happens through working steps with a sponsor and sharing thoughts and experiences with him or her that one might not feel comfortable revealing to a group or in public. Intimacy also comes about through shared experiences.

INTOXICATION

Drunkenness, inebriation, dipsomania. The state of being under the influence of alcohol or other mood-altering drugs; usually used in reference to alcohol consumption. The word "toxic" contained within the word intoxication means "poisonous."

May also refer to being intensely overjoyed or excited to the point that a person becomes irrational; ecstasy, euphoria.

INVENTORY

List, account for, record. In recovery terms, an inventory is a part of both the Fourth and Tenth Step processes, calling for the listing and writing about assets, defects of character, fears, resentments, etc., to discover the exact nature of one's past wrongs/behavior patterns.

Many different acceptable inventory formats are in use in the various fellowships. A sponsor can suggest a format. This part of the program should be done with guidance from a sponsor. The inventory is not done merely to find fault or affix blame, but as an inventory would be done in business—to "uncover, discover, and discard" items that are unusable or unwanted so that they can be replaced with positive qualities.

IRRESPONSIBLE

Negligent, reckless, careless. Displaying lack of accountability or sense of responsibility; unreliable or untrustworthy. Undependable. Considered a character defect.

ISOLATION

Remoteness, seclusion, aloneness. The act or practice of separating from others, remaining alone or apart. Isolation is a major factor in addiction. Active addiction is often marked by using in isolation from others or remaining aloof so one's use of substances or activities is not detected. Isolation may also be the result of paranoia induced by any number of substances.

In recovery, isolation, whether deliberate or unintentional, often precedes a relapse. Failing to avail oneself of the support of the fellowship, skipping or abandoning meetings altogether, or avoiding contact with one's sponsor are all danger signals, and one must monitor one's own behavior to ensure that isolation is not becoming a renewed habit.

ISSUE

Matter, topic, subject. In recovery, a question, concern, or problem. May be a behavior or habit that comes up repeatedly and causes pain and discomfort or keeps an individual from moving on to another level in his or her recovery. Issues may revolve around many topics—abandonment, fear of intimacy, finances, body-image, lifestyle, loss of a loved one—all these (and many more) are issues that can impact one's recovery.

Jj

JACKPOT

Bonanza, top prize, win-all. Originally a positive term from gambling, meaning to win the entire "pot" or "pool." Jackpot has recently acquired an additional negative meaning, often heard during twelve-step meetings, when a speaker describes having landed in a "jam," bind, or crisis that may involve jail time, divorce, or financial hardship, etc.

JEALOUSY

Envy, covetousness, possessiveness. Over-concern for the actions of others and feeling threatened that such actions may deprive one of a need or want. Resentful desire for another's advantages. Unreasonable belief that one's own relationships, possessions, or attributes may be lost or taken by another. Considered a character defect.

JOURNALING

The practice of writing thoughts, feelings, or concerns down on paper (in a journal) in an attempt to work on or process them. Journaling is a beneficial and widely used tool in recovery as an aid to self-knowledge and increasing insight. Continued journaling throughout the course of one's recovery will provide documentary evidence, if any is needed, of the changes one experiences during the journey of recovery.

JOURNEY

Voyage, trip, expedition. A process, rather than an event. Recovery is often compared to a journey, a trip one takes through life, passing through stages along the way, from the depths of despair to the higher ground of a life lived in serenity.

JOY

Happiness, elation, bliss. A life lived in recovery can provide one with the ability to extract joy from simple things, such as family, friendship, and the satisfaction of knowing one is a useful and contributing member of society.

JUDGE/JUDGING

Evaluate/evaluating; decide/deciding; conclude/concluding. Discernment and evaluation are important in recovery in order to make wise decisions, select a sponsor, etc; however, judging others can be problematic in recovery when it becomes the act of finding faults, flaws, or imperfections in others for the purpose of putting them down. One's focus in recovery should be on improving oneself, not on tearing others down. That kind of judging is considered a character defect.

JUDGMENTAL

Hypercritical, condemnatory, disapproving. Engaging in the kind of criticism of others described above, estimating them as "less than," often in order to make oneself feel or seem superior. Considered a character defect.

JUSTIFICATION

Validation, rationalization, excuse. Something, such as a fact or circumstance that is offered as an explanation. Defending oneself. Those in active addiction often use justification as a means to defend their continued use of substances and/or addictive behaviors. Considered a character defect.

Kk

KAFKAESQUE

Relating to the Czech novelist Franz Kafka whose literary works are populated by individuals who are lonely and enigmatic and often find themselves in dark and threatening circumstances. Used at times to refer to surreal or perplexing situations in recovery that members are sometimes confronted with.

KETOSIS

A physical state in which the body produces *ketones* (byproducts created when the body burns fat). This state occurs when people eat fewer carbohydrates than the body needs for fuel; the body then converts fat to energy and weight loss results. Ketosis is seen with a number of popular diets and in anorexia and bulimia.

KEY TAGS

Colored plastic key chains given out at some recovery meetings for various, incremental lengths of time in recovery. Different twelve-step programs have different sets of key tags to designate different lengths of time in recovery; newcomer (24-hours), 30-, 60-, and 90-days, six-, nine-, and eighteen months, plus one year and multiple years. Some fellowships give out plastic or metal "chips" or "tokens," rather than key tags, to celebrate lengths of time in recovery.

KINDNESS

Gentleness, compassion, thoughtfulness. Kindness is a virtue, in recovery as in life, and enables a person in recovery to be available to help others, whether newcomers or old timers, to achieve the common purpose of the twelve-step fellowship.

KNOWLEDGE

Facts, data, awareness. The Eleventh Step refers to gaining knowledge of a higher power's will for one, often gained through prayer and meditation, experience in recovery, through one's own writing, or from interaction with others in recovery.

re•cov•er•y |riˈkəvərē|

L1

LAZINESS

Lethargy, idleness, sloth. Resistant to work or exertion; idle, slow-moving. Considered a character defect.

LEADER(S)

Director(s), chief(s), guide(s). A person who possesses certain qualities that inspire others or invoke enthusiasm; people to whom others look for guidance, direction, hope, inspiration, and comfort, or who provide direction and/or suggestions. Leaders of this type lead by example, not because they hold an official office. May also be the leader or chair of a twelve-step meeting who facilitates the meeting.

Referenced in the Second Tradition of twelve-step programs, which states, ". . . Our leaders are but trusted servants, they do not govern." This tradition cautions members who are considered leaders that they lead by example rather than directing or acting on self-will.

LEADERSHIP

The act or practice of being a leader; the act of behaving in such a way as to provide direction, guidance, or inspiration that other people choose to follow.

LEGAL DRUGS

Prescribed medications and over-the-counter medication (OTC medication). Although legal, these substances can be mind- and mood-altering. Those in recovery need to practice extreme caution when taking prescribed or OTC medication and stay in close contact with their sponsor, especially if the prescribed medication is an opioid or painkiller.

Alcohol is considered a legal drug.

LETTING GO

The practice of turning a problem over to one's higher power. This can be described as practicing the Third Step. "Let go and let God," is one expression of this principle used in recovery.

LIABILITIES

Weaknesses, problems, burdens. Actions, attitudes, or behaviors a person resorts to in addiction or in addictive behavior that keep him or her separated from others or from his or her higher power. In recovery, liabilities may also be referred to as character defects and are often identified in Step Four and addressed in Steps Six and Seven.

LIMITATION(S)

Restriction(s), constraint(s), inadequacy(ies). Reaching the end of one's abilities or capacity. A person in recovery who is spiritually fit, that is, practicing twelve-step recovery in all his or her affairs, typically has very few limitations on what he or she can do or where he or she can go in recovery.

LISTEN

Take note, to hear, pay attention. An active part of the communication process between two or more people takes place when one listens to what another is saying and processes and interprets that information. In early recovery, newcomers especially are advised to "learn to listen, then listen to learn."

LITERATURE

Writing, text, prose. In twelve-step programs, the term "recovery literature" refers to books, workbooks, information pamphlets, or service manuals that have been approved by the World or General Service Organizations that have to do with the nature of addiction and recovery. Many people in recovery who live in remote locations where there are few meetings or who are incarcerated, hospitalized, or institutionalized rely on the message contained in the basic texts of their fellowships for comfort and support when another person in recovery is not available.

LITERATURE DISTRIBUTION SUBCOMMITTEE

A number of twelve-step fellowships have a literature distribution subcommittee that takes and fulfills literature orders from local groups. This subcommittee is typically part of the area service committee. This is terminology specific to the service structure found in most twelve-step fellowships.

LONELINESS

Isolation, aloneness, friendlessness. A painful and unpleasant feeling, common among persons in active addiction, and sometimes among those in recovery. Usually a deep feeling of sequestration, isolation, or seclusion due either to actual physical separation from others or from a feeling of being disconnected from others on an emotional, mental, or spiritual level.

LONG-TERM RECOVERY

Term used to help people understand that recovery means a person is no longer using alcohol or other drugs. This term is an effort on behalf of a number of recovery advocacy organizations to destigmatize the disease of addiction since the word "addict" and/or "alcoholic" is often viewed negatively by the general public. Also can help people understand that there is more to recovery than not using alcohol or other drugs, and that part of recovery is creating a better life.

LOST

Missing, gone, disoriented. In the metaphysical or philosophical sense, to not know where one belongs or where one is going. Mentally, to be confused or disoriented. Spiritually, a feeling of being out of place, different from others, a beat behind, or disconnected from a higher power; not knowing what will happen, not being familiar with practices, customs, etc. The feeling of being lost is best overcome by increased participation in one's twelve-step fellowship, by ongoing step work, meeting attendance, and service work.

LOVE

Devotion, care, concern. The willing extension of one's self for the spiritual, emotional, mental, and physical betterment of another. The love that is felt and practiced in twelve-step fellowships is real and enduring. It is the sort of "brotherly" or "sisterly" love that is expressed in very practical ways—by calling others on the phone, by giving a ride to a newcomer who's without a car, by inviting a person who is alone to share a meal, etc. This love is the missing ingredient in the lives of most persons in active addiction, and may be replaced in full by membership in a twelve-step fellowship.

LUST

Intense sexual hunger, longing or desire, particularly when unaccompanied by love. May also refer to enthusiastic zeal. When focused on sexual hunger or longing, it is considered a character defect.

LYING

Deceiving, being untruthful, telling falsehoods. Lying may be by omission (not telling something or not telling *all* about something) or by commission (actually creating false information). Active addiction is a life built on lying. Considered a character defect.

Recovery is a life built on honesty—with oneself, a higher power, and others.

re·cov·er·y |riˈkəvərē|

Mm

MAGICAL THINKING

A type of "relapse-prone" thinking. In this type of thinking, those in twelve-step programs may imagine that using again will solve any difficulties they may be having in recovery, forgetting that it was active addiction that led to most of their problems in the first place.

MAINTAIN

Preserve, uphold, continue. Regular effort one must expend in order to continue on a current path. To do the work necessary on an ongoing basis in order to continue to grow in one's recovery.

MAINTENANCE

The process of preserving, upholding, or continuing something. Expending effort on a regular basis to maintain one's recovery. To participate regularly in the recovery process and all that entails; attending meetings, making sponsor contact, reading recommended literature, writing and working steps, being of service, etc.

Also a term used in the treatment of opiate (heroin) addiction in which a person is provided with a medical prescription for opiate substitutes such as methadone or buprenorphine.

MANIPULATION

Exploitation, handling, coercing. The act or practice of influencing others' behavior by intimidating, bullying, lying, or pressuring them. The state of being manipulated. Shrewd or devious management usually for one's own advantage. Not necessarily violent or overt. Considered a character defect.

MARAJUANA ANONYMOUS (MA)

This twelve-step fellowship, founded in 1989, helps people recover from marijuana addiction. The only requirement for membership is a desire to stop using marijuana. *Life with Hope* is the title of MA's recovery book.

MATERIALISM

Avariciousness, greediness, covetousness. A great or excessive regard for worldly concerns. Placing physical possessions ahead of spiritual growth. The belief that physical well-being and worldly possessions constitute the greatest good and highest value in life, usually at the expense of the spiritual. Considered by many to be a character defect.

MEAN

Unkind, cruel, malicious. The state of being selfish, stingy, hostile, or aggressive to another. Spiteful or callous. Unusually or excessively marked by animosity. Considered a character defect.

MEDICATION

A medicinal substance, drug, medicine. In recovery terms, any medicine prescribed by a medical professional legally authorized to write prescriptions. Doctors, psychiatrists, and nurse-practitioners may prescribe medication to treat illnesses, ailments, or injuries. Medication may either be prescribed to alleviate symptoms or to cure an illness.

MEDITATE/MEDITATION

Reflect, contemplate, ponder. To attempt to focus the mind on one thought, to relax the mind. A centering, peaceful, serene, or grounding exercise. There are many different meditation techniques; meditation is a very personal process, unique for each person. Some people use breathing exercises, visualizations, mantras (repeated words or phrases), or other specific techniques, while others may simply sit in silence and attempt to concentrate on their own breath. While there are many different traditions and programs that teach specific practices, ultimately, it is something that is adapted by the individual to fit his or her needs.

An essential element of the Eleventh Step as members deepen their connection with their higher power, as in "Sought through prayer and meditation to improve our conscious contact with God. . . ."

MEDITATION BOOK

A daily reinforcement of recovery in a condensed, easy-to-read format. These books give a recovering person a positive thought to focus on as they go about their recovery each day. There are many different types of meditation books, geared toward particular issues or groups, including addicts, alcoholics, compulsive gamblers, men, women, codependents, adult children of alcoholics, those suffering from mental illness, abuse survivors, etc.

MEETING

Assembly, gathering, get-together. Two or more people coming together for the purpose of recovery from their addiction constitutes a recovery meeting. A setting in which people can meet for the purpose of sharing experience, strength, and hope with one another. Twelve-step meetings take place at regularly scheduled locations and times and are listed in a schedule/meeting list, and are usually populated with members who attend on a regular basis and perform service commitments that ensure the meeting is run smoothly and properly. Formats vary by program and community, but follow a basic pattern.

Common formats include: speaker meetings, open discussion, literature studies, step studies, topic discussion, etc. Some meetings may be more specialized within a particular twelve-step program.

MEETING ETIQUETTE (See section on Meeting and Fellowship Etiquette, page 217.)

Decorum, manners, protocol. The etiquette, or acceptable behavior, for persons attending meetings varies in different twelve-step programs and among various groups and meetings within each particular program; however, certain activities are universally accepted while others are universally discouraged. Examples of discouraged behaviors may include "cross-talking," talking with one's neighbors, using communication devices like cell phones during meetings, bringing children or others to a closed meeting, or leaving one's seat noisily and/or repeatedly. Etiquette can be easily learned by using common sense and by visiting a variety of different meetings while observing what is acceptable behavior there.

MEMBER

Constituent, associate, affiliate. One who belongs. A person who identifies as being a part of a twelve-step program. The Third Tradition in various programs states that the "only requirement for membership is a desire to stop" using, drinking, or participating in certain activities, but it does not insist that one must be clean/sober/abstinent before becoming a member or even after attending several meetings.

MEMBERSHIP

The state of belonging-to, participating-in, or signing-up for a group, fraternity, fellowship etc., such as a twelve-step fellowship. Requirements and stipulations for membership depend on the type of group, but it is generally accepted within most twelve-step fellowships that membership starts when one says one is a member; "the only requirement for membership" being the desire to enter recovery.

MENTAL ILLNESS

Madness, insanity, psychosis. Lack of mental health or clarity, mental suffering. Mental conditions such as: clinical depression, schizophrenia, dementia, etc. that go beyond the scope of twelve-step programs, which are designed to deal with the disease of addiction, which may or may not be considered a form of mental illness in itself.

Mental illnesses usually require attention from a medical doctor or psychiatrist, and this need is recognized and stated in most twelve-step literature. The Twelve Steps are an effective treatment for addiction, and though they may be helpful in ameliorating a person's mental illness, they are not a substitute for medical or psychiatric treatment.

MESSAGE

Communication, meaning, epistle. The message of recovery is the mission statement of twelve-step fellowships that "there is a solution," and recovery is possible through working the Twelve Steps.

MIDDLE-CIRCLE BEHAVIORS

In sex and love addiction recovery, "middle-circle behaviors" are behaviors that may be safe but that might under some circumstances lead back to "inner-circle" behaviors, which would constitute a relapse. These behaviors differ from person to person in recovery, and are worked out with guidance from a sponsor.

MIRACLE

Phenomenon, marvel, wonder. Any event apparently beyond human powers and ordinary understanding of the laws of nature. Any happening so unusual as to have been thought impossible, such as a mother suddenly having the strength to lift a car that had run over her child, to an addict getting one day clean. Usually attributed to some sort of divine providence or intervention from a higher power. It is a miracle of recovery when someone suffering from addiction can get one day of recovery because he or she could not stop using addictively.

MODERATION

Temperance, restraint, self-control. Balance between extremes. To engage in an activity within limitations, not acting or doing something to excess. Twelve-step recovery from alcohol, drugs, or gambling does not teach moderation—it is based on abstinence.

However, recovery from certain "process" addictions, like compulsive eating, codependence, or sex, calls for moderation, rather than abstinence. Eating, relationships, and sex are necessary life functions/activities that have been carried to an extreme in addiction—to abstain from them would not be considered healthy.

MONEY ISSUES

Problems relating to money; financial issues; whether related to over-spending, under-earning, or failure to establish or follow a budget or pay bills, can affect a person's recovery, which is why being a productive member of society, working and being self-supporting is so important.

MOOD-ALTERING

Anything that changes or alters one's disposition or frame of mind. Refers to any drug, including alcohol, consumed by an individual to effect a change in, or alter, consciousness, feelings, or emotional state; may include other substances or activities (manifestations of addiction) that a person might use to change the way he or she feels, such as food, caffeine, nicotine, shopping, sex, etc.

MORALS

Values, ethics, principles. A code of beliefs influencing a person's own behavior. Morals relate to a personal understanding of right and wrong. Although each individual person must develop his or her own particular moral code, there are generally accepted moral conventions that have throughout time been consistent across all cultures, e.g., that it is wrong to kill or steal from others. In recovery, an addict discovers his or her own personal morals: what is right and wrong for him or her through working the Twelve Steps.

MORAL INVENTORY

The listing of past actions, resentments, assets and liabilities in an attempt to determine the exact nature of wrong and right behavior and to reveal character defects that one will ask a higher power to remove in the Seventh Step. Part of the Fourth Step in a twelve-step recovery program.

MORBID

Gloomy, melancholic, dark. Psychologically unhealthy or unwholesome. Characterized by preoccupation with unwholesome thoughts or feelings. Gruesome; grisly. Considered a character defect.

Nn

NAR-ANON

A worldwide twelve-step fellowship whose aim is to assist family members and loved ones to recover from the disease of addiction in their family. Nar-Anon has meetings in the US, Canada, and other countries.

NARCOTICS ANONYMOUS (NA)

A twelve-step recovery program that addresses the disease of addiction. To emphasize that it is a "we" program, and to differentiate from AA's Twelve Steps, the first eleven steps begin with the word "We" and reference to alcohol is changed to "our addiction" in the First Step. The only requirement for membership is a "desire to stop using." While there is no direct reference to specific substances, it is stated in the fellowship's literature that "NA is a nonprofit fellowship or society of men and women for whom drugs had become a major problem."

NA was formed in July 1953 in California, with literature translated into thirty-six languages, and meetings in more than 134 countries around the world. The founder of Narcotics Anonymous is considered to be an addict named Jimmy K. The fellowship's recovery text is titled *Narcotics Anonymous*.

NATURE

Environment, life, character. The natural world or the basic, elemental character and temperament of a person or a thing. The nature of something is what it *is* fundamentally. Discovering one's own nature would include discovering the causes or roots of problems that are not attributable to any outside person or any event, but that are characteristic solely of oneself.

Addressed specifically in Step Five as one admits to ". . . God, ourselves, and another human being the exact nature of our wrongs."

NAWS

Narcotics Anonymous World Services, or NAWS, is the non-profit corporation for the fellowship of Narcotics Anonymous. The World Service Office (WSO) is the primary headquarters, located in Chatsworth, California. WSO is an office where Narcotics Anonymous literature can be purchased and is the hub for fellowship development services and communication.

NAWSO

Nicotine Anonymous World Service Office began in 1986. Its officers and leadership ensure that the fellowship adheres to the steps and traditions, publish NicA literature such as books and brochures that define its recovery program, and attend to Nicotine Anonymous business affairs.

NEEDY

Deprived, needing affection, distressed. Emotional state of exhibiting an intense need for love or other emotional support. In recovery, this definition is considered a character defect.

Also refers to someone who is impoverished, destitute, or poverty-stricken.

NEGATIVE

Pessimistic, unenthusiastic, downbeat. Indicating opposition or resistance. Having no positive features. Exhibiting features that are not positive or constructive. Being constantly negative is considered a character defect.

NEWCOMER(S)

A person (or persons) in early recovery. There is no specific length of time one is considered a newcomer—it varies and is more a function of immersion in the program and one's progress through the steps. The main focus during early recovery is on such activities as meeting attendance on a daily basis, reading recovery literature, building a relationship with a sponsor and a support group, joining a home group and possibly taking a service commitment; all referred to as "building a foundation."

NICOTINE ANONYMOUS (NicA)

Nicotine Anonymous is a twelve-step fellowship for those seeking freedom from nicotine addiction, including those using cessation programs and nicotine-withdrawal aids. NicA began in Southern California in 1982 and today has over 500 meetings worldwide. Its recovery text is titled *Nicotine Anonymous, The Book.*

NINTH STEP

From the Twelve Steps (Step Nine). The Ninth Step requires the recovering person to make amends to all people he or she has harmed, except when doing so would cause further damage to the injured party or others. One may make amends directly or indirectly. Paying back owed money would be an example of making a direct amend. Volunteering at a day care center might constitute indirect amends for having abandoned a child one is presently unable to contact or care for. The guidance of a sponsor is helpful and often recommended when making amends.

NINTH TRADITION

From the Twelve Traditions (Tradition Nine). A guideline for twelve-step programs stating that twelve-step groups and members should never be under external management or control (". . . ought never be organized"), but that those groups may form service boards and committees that are directly responsible to the groups the boards and committees serve.

NON-AFFILIATION

Not closely connected; to have no direct association, in name or function, with an organization, group, association, company, or individual outside of the twelve-step program, such as a treatment center or hospital, although the twelve-step program may cooperate with such institutions or hold meetings on its premises.

NON-DISCRIMINATION

To not exclude or not include members because of some factor such as race, creed, religion, lack of religion, sexual orientation, or any held values or opinions. Twelve-step programs welcome any person who has the desire to stop using/acting out/etc. on his or her manifestation of addiction regardless of his or her background, social status, etc.

NON-PROFESSIONAL

A person (worker) who is not paid to provide counsel, nor are they a doctor or therapist bound by the Hippocratic oath. A person who is not a professional in a specific field; without licensure or degree. In twelve-step programs, even if a person is a professional in his or her private life, he or she does not identify as a professional, but rather as a member of the program. He or she does not give advice to sponsees in a professional capacity either, but merely as a fellowship member.

NOSINESS

Over-inquisitiveness, snooping, prying. Given to excessive prying into the affairs of others. Considered a character defect.

Oo

OBSESSION

Fascination, passion, mania. An intense, insistent, constant drive, need, or fixation (fixed idea), desire, all-one-can-think-of, constant thinking about a specific topic, idea, problem, person, or situation to the exclusion of all else. Continual thoughts of using drugs or acting out on a behavior. An intense feeling that one must use drugs or act out on a behavior to satisfy the obsession, no matter what the consequences are. A primary component of the disease of addiction.

OBSESSIVE COMPULSIVE DISORDER (OCD)

Obsessive Compulsive Disorder is a type of anxiety disorder, and as such, untreated OCD sufferers may self-medicate with alcohol or other drugs in an effort to find relief. Like those suffering with addiction, OCD sufferers experience obsession—repeated, obtrusive, unwelcome thoughts—and compulsions—the need to perform certain rituals to reduce their anxiety. OCD can be treated with a combination of therapy and medication. It is not addiction *per se,* although addiction does contain elements of obsession and compulsion.

OLD TIMER

A recovering person with significant clean time/sobriety/abstinence/
recovery; specific time depends on geographic location, particular twelve-
step program, and on the general "age" of the local recovery community.
An old timer is a person with significant experience in a twelve-step
program, who has spent a great deal of time abstaining from a substance
or behavior and living "life on life's terms," free from active addiction.
People with substantial clean time/sobriety/abstinence/recovery who
have more experience dealing with life situations and have a greater
distance between themselves and active using than newcomers.

OMNIPOTENT

Invincible, all-powerful, almighty, supreme. This word is usually
associated with the God of Western religion, and many in twelve-step
recovery understand their higher power to be omnipotent. Along with
omnipotence, the higher power is also considered to possess omniscience
(all knowledge), and omnipresence (universal presence), etc.

ON-LINE GAMERS ANONYMOUS (OLGA)

A twelve-step self-help fellowship that helps individuals to recover from
the problems caused by excessive game playing, whether it be computer,
video, console, or online. OLGA was founded in May 2002 by Elizabeth
Woolley whose son, Shawn, committed suicide as a probable result of
being addicted to one of the online games.

OPEN MEETINGS

Twelve-step meetings that welcome persons who are not members of
that particular fellowship, including family members or members of the
general public who may be interested in seeing how the meetings are run
or how the program works. Sometimes a person who is not quite ready
to enter a twelve-step program as a member will attend open meetings to
"test the waters."

OPEN-MINDEDNESS

A non-judgmental attitude, tolerance, impartiality. The quality of accepting others' right to their own feelings and opinions, listening respectfully to other opinions, ideas, beliefs, or suggestions, and being open to the possibility that those ideas have merit. A willingness to listen to another person in recovery and attempt to hear what that person has to share. The humility necessary to listen to opposing points of view. Considered a spiritual principle.

OPINION

Estimation, belief, judgment. A judgment or personal, subjective analysis of a topic, issue, situation, etc. What a person or group may feel, believe, or value about a certain situation, topic, etc. Opinions are often based on feelings, beliefs, or fears, or on past experiences rather than on knowledge or facts.

As related to the Tenth Tradition, twelve-step fellowships have "no opinion on outside issues." This ensures that the fellowship will not be drawn into any outside controversies, therefore protecting not only the reputation of the fellowship, but enabling it to maintain its primary purpose—recovery.

ORDER

Stability, organization, tidiness. Also refers to sequence, ranking, classification, as in the saying, "the steps are in order for a reason," which implies that it is wise to finish one step before moving on to the next. For example, those who are new to recovery have a tendency to immediately want to make amends or to tell others that they are sorry for past wrongs—when making amends actually means putting things right, and not just saying "sorry." Most people in early recovery are very sorry and remorseful, but have no idea how to go about making true amends, which may be why making amends is Step Nine in the process.

OUTER-CIRCLE BEHAVIORS

In sex and love addiction recovery, "outer-circle behaviors" are behaviors that the recovering sex addict may engage in without fear of a relapse; they may include non-sexual hugging, as in greeting, a kiss on the cheek for a friend, or even sexual activity with a spouse or longtime partner who is aware and supportive of the sex addict's recovery program.

OUTSIDE ENTERPRISES

Enterprises are businesses, business activities aimed at profit, or organizations. "Outside enterprises" are organizations, associations, companies, or political entities that are not connected or affiliated with twelve-step programs. Ideally, twelve-step program members should not share about/discuss politics, religion, or other "off-topic" subjects at meetings, but should confine their comments to the common problem that the meeting addresses, rather than "outside enterprises." Fellowship members should never exploit their program membership for financial gain, e.g., to promote their own outside businesses.

OUTSIDE ISSUE(S)

Matters or concerns outside the realm of addiction and recovery. There are differing opinions about what these issues might be. Many believe that mentioning other fellowships (such as by discussing drugs in an AA meeting or alcohol in a GA meeting), talking about politics, religion, the need for medication in recovery, etc. might fall into this category. Others believe this term refers to the need for the twelve-step fellowship as a whole to avoid endorsing or expressing any opinion on issues that do not concern the program itself. As a general rule, especially for a new member, anything that affects the individual personally or his or her ability to recover is not an outside issue.

Typically relates to the Tenth Tradition.

OVEREATERS ANONYMOUS (OA)

A twelve-step fellowship whose primary focus is to help people recover from compulsive eating. OA is not about weight loss, weight gain, binge eating, or bulimia. It is not about obesity or diets. It addresses physical, emotional, and spiritual well-being. Its recovery text is called *Overeaters Anonymous.*

OA was cofounded by Rozanne S and Jo S in 1960. These two members, along with another compulsive overeater, Bernice S, held the first OA meeting in Los Angeles, California. Today there are more than 6,500 OA groups in more than seventy-five countries, with approximately 55,000 members worldwide.

OVERLY ANALYTICAL

Excessively critical, methodical, obsessive, to the detriment of one's program of recovery, which is not solely an intellectual exercise; it involves the physical, emotional, mental, and spiritual in balance. Considered a character defect.

Pp

PAIN

Soreness, aching, hurt. Suffering, whether physical, mental, or emotional, from an affliction or due to having been hurt or injured. Anguish over a given situation or set of circumstances. Emotional pain is believed to underlie active addiction as much as physical pain, although persons suffering physical pain for extended periods of time (chronic pain) are in danger of becoming addicted to opioid painkillers or of "self-medicating" with alcohol or other drugs and may need to enter their own program of recovery to address both their pain issues and their addiction. Pain is a part of life for everyone. People in recovery learn to accept pain without the use of chemicals for relief.

PARADOX

Contradiction, inconsistency, irony. Two ideas that in theory cannot coexist or two juxtaposed concepts that appear opposite; expressed in twelve-step quotes such as "surrender to win."

PARALLEL

Corresponding, equivalent, running-alongside. A resemblance or congruence. Railroad tracks are often cited as an example of things that are parallel.

PARANOID

Fearful, mistrustful, suspicious. Suffering from fear of real or imaginary situations or enemies or feeling that other people are out to harm one. Can be and is often a result of excessive use of mind- and mood-altering chemicals or extreme trauma or abuse. A fear or expectation that one is going to be hurt or deceived by others; a profound distrust of other people, or feeling as if one is being conspired against. Connected to self-centeredness and self-obsession. Considered a character defect.

PASSIVE

Submissive, unreceptive, inert. Receiving or subjected to an action without responding or initiating an action in return. Accepting or submitting to a situation or to the unwelcome action of another without objection, resistance, or verbal complaint. Considered a character defect.

PATHWAYS

In recovery terms, pathways relate to and focus on the solutions, strategies, and experiences that contribute to recovery and are further enhanced through the recovery process. Effective pathways to recovery can be medical, public health, faith, or social support approaches that improve personal well-being as well as the lives of children, families, and communities. There is no one pathway to recovery and the journey can be guided by religious faith, spiritual experience, and/or secular teachings.

PATIENCE

Staying power, endurance, lack of complaint. A spiritual principle. The state of being tolerant with and of others, the ability to wait, the ability to allow time to pass before making a decision or taking action. Doing the footwork necessary for a result without expecting immediate gratification. Allowing another person to experience his or her feelings; it can be a form or demonstration of love. A person practicing patience does not react in anger when something does not turn out as he or she may have desired.

PATTERN(S)

Model, prototype, plan used in making things. A system of behavior or a series of behaviors that lead to similar outcomes. A *modus operandi*, hidden agenda, habitual behavior, or chronic, repeated reaction to different life events or situations. A person in recovery usually will uncover behavior patterns after completing a Fourth Step inventory. It is important to identify patterns that led to active addiction and develop healthy patterns that can aid one's recovery.

PEACE

Tranquility, calm, serenity. A state of harmony, quiet, an absence of crisis or chaos. Existence in a state of acceptance. The ability to live "life on life's terms" with some ease and comfort. The opposite of chaos or turmoil, of being uncomfortable, feeling in danger, or experiencing stress or anxiety.

PEER PRESSURE

Perceived pressure or coercion to take part in an activity that is exerted by a person's equals, colleagues, cohorts. Adolescents are famously prone to peer pressure, but it exists at every stage of life. Friends, family, siblings, schoolmates, and co-workers and friends in the fellowship are examples of peers. Peer pressure is something individuals face from "people, places, and things," which may create roadblocks to recovery. Alternatively, peer pressure can be positive; a person in recovery who surrounds himself or herself with clean/sober/abstinent/recovering friends will feel positive peer pressure to stay in recovery.

PEOPLE, PLACES, AND THINGS

The persons, locations, and items associated with an individual's using, drinking, or participating in addictive behaviors; may include the physical location where drug use or addictive behavior occurred and/or the activities, paraphernalia, etc. that are associated with active addiction. Also referred to as "old playmates, playgrounds, and playthings."

PEOPLE-PLEASING

Deriving one's value and worth from the approval of others. Performing an action in order to please another, rather than out of an intrinsic desire or interest. Considered a character defect.

PERCEPTION

Awareness, insight, discernment. The way a person looks at things. Past experiences, knowledge, feelings, judgments, attitudes, etc. that affect one's interpretation of a given situation. In recovery, it is important for an individual to check his or her perception of events against that of trusted friends or sponsors.

PERFECTION

Flawlessness, rightness, excellence. The state of being without blemishes, defects, or shortcomings. To arrive at a state at which one does not require any further work, recovery, transformation, or change. Recovery is a state of "progress, not perfection."

PERSEVERANCE

Resolve, firmness, steadfastness. Continuous, steady action and/or belief, often in spite of great difficulty. A spiritual principle that calls for remaining on the path of recovery through difficult, unfortunate, or painful times. Staying in recovery and continuing to work through tumultuous situations, illnesses, relationships ending, etc.

PERSONAL INVENTORY

Also known as a "Fourth-Step Inventory," "Moral Inventory," and "Tenth-Step Inventory." The major focus of the Fourth and Tenth Step processes.

The Fourth Step inventory is a formal and considered undertaking. This step should be worked with the guidance of a sponsor, and as the language of the step indicates, should be both "searching and fearless." One's own history is examined and listed honestly.

When used in reference to the Tenth Step, taking personal inventory consists of reviewing one's day to discover continuing patterns of selfishness, resentfulness, dishonesty, and fear. It is suggested that this step be taken nightly, before retiring, as part of one's reflection on one's behavior and feelings that day, in order to enhance the maintenance of one's spiritual fitness.

PERSONALITY

Individuality, persona, character. The collection of physical expressions and character traits, including assets and defects, a person possesses, as well as the attitude he or she expresses toward life. The unique expression of one's nature and character in the way one may dress, speak, or carry him- or herself.

PERSPECTIVE

Perception, outlook, point of view. A particular view of a situation or a way of seeing things, whether in a positive or negative manner. May change if new information is gathered or if viewed in light of alternative considerations or from a transcended or enlightened point of view.

PITFALLS

Snare, downside, hazard. An unexpected danger, usually as the result of one's not being cognizant of one's surroundings or situation. Examples in recovery may include unhealthy relationships, living beyond one's means, and/or becoming too involved in service or some other aspect of the program and getting out of balance with the rest of the program.

PLAN(S)

Program(s), scheme(s), method(s). A set of ideas or suggestions as to a course of action. May be a set of goals or objectives or a path to achieve those goals or objectives. Setting goals, making arrangements, or making a commitment to perform an activity with another person.

PLASTIC SURGERY ADDICTION

As the cost of procedures has made cosmetic plastic surgery more affordable to the average person, the number of patients who seem to become "addicted" to cosmetic surgery is growing. Many of these individuals suffer from a condition known as Body Dysmorphic Disorder, a psychological disorder characterized by an obsessive preoccupation with one or more of their own physical features, which they believe are deformed or particularly socially unacceptable. Such individuals seek out numerous treatments and surgeries to rid themselves of the "offending" characteristic. The relief they obtain is transitory at best, as the "problem" is one of low self-esteem. No specific twelve-step fellowships yet address this problem, but Cognitive-Behavioral Therapy offers some help and the condition is attracting researchers.

POLICY/POLICIES

Strategy/strategies, rule(s), guideline(s). The parameters within which the business of an organization such as a twelve-step fellowship is conducted. Used during business meetings, subcommittee meetings, etc. Policies are suggested and voted on by the group (group conscience). Often based on the collective experience of what has worked well in the past.

POTENTIAL

Probable, likely, possible. Also refers to the level to which someone or something could possibly rise, goals that one can achieve, or the abilities one has within him- or herself that are yet to be realized. An individual's potential is the unrealized capability that he or she hopes to realize in and as a result of recovery.

POWER

Energy, force, control. The ability to generate action, a source of strength, vigor, or ability, as in "the power to carry that out" in Step Eleven.

POWER GREATER THAN OURSELVES

A benevolent force outside of oneself that has more strength than one possesses. A "higher power" or power other than a person that can effect a restoration to sanity. A "power greater than ourselves" is first mentioned in Step Two of the Twelve Steps. The concept of a power greater than oneself is key to working a twelve-step program of recovery, is very personal, and evolves over time.

POWERLESS

Ineffective, immobilized, defenseless. The state of being without power, particularly regarding the disease of addiction. Having no control over a situation, being unable to control behavior or actions, e.g., unable to control the use of alcohol or other drugs, behaviors, thoughts, feelings, etc. Having no control over people, places, and things.

As related to recovery, the primary concept of Step One in which a person admits he or she is powerless over whatever manifestation of addiction he or she is addressing. Without this critical admission, accepting that one has the disease of addiction, and surrendering to the principles of the Twelve Steps, one rarely will stay in recovery.

PRACTICAL APPLICATION

Actively putting to a special use. Putting a plan into action, applying what has been learned. Taking concrete and defined steps toward a stated goal to achieve a particular outcome; that outcome may include being free from active addiction. In recovery, putting the steps into action in one's life is an example of practical application of the program.

PRACTICE

Carry out, perform, apply. Engage in an activity or task to increase one's proficiency at that activity or task or to prepare for an upcoming activity or task of increased difficulty. Step Twelve states ". . . to practice these principles in all our affairs," which is a direction to persons in the fellowships to live the Twelve Steps in every aspect of their lives to the best of their abilities in order to enjoy long-lasting recovery.

PRAYER

Entreaty, appeal, plea. The act of communication with a higher power or God of one's understanding. May take many forms, formal or informal, with ritual, or through simple communication in a conversational manner, in solitude or in communion with others, in any body posture, including on one's knees. This practice can change, evolve, and grow over time, as one's understanding of recovery changes and grows.

PREDECESSOR(S)

Forerunner, ancestor, precursor. One who came before. The first people or group to do something; pioneers. People involved in the beginning of a movement. Used in recovery terms, relates to the individuals who founded the twelve-step programs and created the model for today's recovery programs. The authors of recovery literature, service manuals, etc. who gave of themselves in order for the fellowships to survive and flourish.

PREJUDICE

Bias, narrow-mindedness, bigotry. An adverse judgment or opinion formed beforehand or without knowledge or examination of the facts. A preconceived preference or idea. Irrational suspicion or hatred of a particular group, race, religion, etc. Considered a character defect.

PRESTIGE

Honor, regard, high esteem. In recovery, self-important concern about prestige can draw one's attention away from the primary purpose of a twelve-step program and prevent one from developing the humility needed for the surrender that is a part of the twelve-step recovery process. The Sixth Tradition cautions members specifically about being diverted from their primary purpose by "problems of money, property, or prestige."

PRIDE

Arrogance, conceit, smugness. Can be a character defect when it sets one apart from others as being better than them. But pride can be a positive feeling of accomplishment, as in taking pride in one's work, actions, family, etc. One avoids feeling too "proud" of one's recovery, as this can often lead to delusions of self-sufficiency or self-reliance, which frequently lead to feelings of invulnerability, of not needing the program, and often, relapse.

PRIMARY PURPOSE

The priority, the first task, the basic focus. In twelve-step programs, "to carry the message to the (addict, alcoholic, compulsive gambler, etc.) who still suffers" is the primary purpose. The message is that recovery is possible; that the program, if followed, will lead to a life of recovery.

PRINCIPLES (SPIRITUAL PRINCIPLES)

Ethics, morality, values. Referring to spiritual principles found within the steps, which form a code of conduct by which to live. Positive actions recovering people strive to live by that are found embedded in the Twelve Steps, Twelve Traditions, and Twelve Concepts. Examples include: hope, faith, trust, patience, courage, perseverance, humility, honesty, willingness, open-mindedness, service, tolerance, compassion, and anonymity, which is described as the "spiritual foundation" of all the Twelve Traditions.

PRIORITY

Importance, primacy, main concern. Something requiring immediate attention. The present matter or the issue that must be addressed before other things. In recovery, the action or task that comes before all others, and upon which everything else, such as, work, returning to or furthering one's education, relationships, children's demands, etc depends. Most twelve-step programs encourage their members to make their recovery a priority.

PRIVACY

Confidentiality, discretion, solitude. The keeping of possessions, thoughts, or valuables secure or private. Keeping intimate personal information secure. Privacy is not the same as isolation. It is appropriate for some conversations and activities to be carried on in privacy; however, in recovery one learns the difference between maintaining a healthy and respectful privacy and an unhealthy isolation. A sponsor keeps the sponsee's confidences; this builds trust and is about privacy; it is not the same as keeping secrets, which is negative and unhealthy.

Keeping one's anonymity in public is an example of healthy privacy.

PRIVILEGE

Advantage, license, benefit. Something not guaranteed or something one does not necessarily have a right to. A "perk" or benefit that comes as the result of performance or one's actions. Privileges must be earned by behavior; they may be granted or withheld based on one's actions.

PROCESS

Method, course of action, procedure. Continuing development requiring many changes; involving many components and variables. Refers to the idea that recovery does not happen overnight, instantly, or quickly. The position that a person in recovery will never be "fully" recovered and that recovery is an ongoing course of action or development. The process of recovery is said to take place in stages, first physically, then mentally/emotionally, and finally spiritually. Relapse is believed to occur in the opposite order; first spiritually, then emotionally/mentally, and then physically."

PROCESS ADDICTION

A wide variety of mood-altering behaviors and activities that can create cycles of obsessive thinking and compulsive behaving that characterize addiction. Typically does not involve the ingestion of substances/chemicals. Behaviors and activities commonly considered to be process addictions include, gambling, shopping or spending, exercise, sex, work, video games, and the Internet to name but a few.

There are a number of twelve-step fellowships that exist to support those who suffer from this form of addiction.

PROCRASTINATION

Delaying, postponing, deferring. Refers to an action that needs to be or should be taken. Avoiding action because of subconscious fear or because of laziness, time constraints, financial situations, etc. Delaying an action by conscious choice. Looking for alternatives to an unpleasant or undesirable task or allowing oneself to be distracted by miscellaneous and unnecessary tasks before finally doing what is required. Considered a character defect.

PROGRESSION

Advance, development, evolution. Continuous forward movement. To continue on a particular track, be it negative or positive. In active addiction, progression may mean needing more of a particular substance or activity to achieve the same effect. Also refers to the accumulation of the negative consequences of addiction. The disease of addiction is often referred to as "chronic, progressive, and fatal" if left untreated.

In recovery, the Twelve Steps follow a positive progression, each step building upon the last, as the person in recovery learns more skills to cope with situations the longer he or she stays clean/sober/abstinent.

PROJECTION

Prediction, forecast, assessment. In recovery, often refers to worrying about situations or events that may not occur or fear of a specific outcome. May also refer to the psychological defense mechanism of projection whereby one's own thoughts, motivations, attitudes, etc. are attributed to others, i.e., "projected onto others."

Associated with thinking of negative outcomes or having expectations. Thinking the worst thing that could happen, will happen. A mindset that assumes horrible things will occur.

PROMISE(S)

Vow, commitment, agreement. A guarantee of something to come when directions or suggestions are followed in a twelve-step program. The Big Book of Alcoholics Anonymous contains twelve statements that have come to be known as "The Promises," which outline what spiritual benefits one can expect to achieve through working the Twelve Steps. Several other fellowships, such as Overeaters Anonymous, Emotions Anonymous, and Debtors Anonymous, also have promises. In Narcotics Anonymous there is one promise, "freedom from active addiction," if a recovering addict works the Twelve Steps.

PROMOTION

Endorsement, advertisement, support. The practice of claiming superiority of a product or service, putting one method or system above others. In the Eleventh Tradition, the value of promotion is contrasted with the value of attraction; the tradition asserts that twelve-step fellowships will not proselytize or attempt to gain members through advertising or promotion, but rather that the individual members' actions as program members in recovery should be the thing that attracts new members.

PROMPTLY

Right away, as soon as possible, done at once. Part of Step Ten: ". . . and when we were wrong, promptly admitted it." Fellowship members review their behavior continually, and when they realize they have wronged or hurt another (whether that person is a program member or not), they admit their wrong and make amends to that person immediately.

PROVEN

Verified, confirmed, established. Shown to be true. A fact or statement that has been demonstrated with examples, such as, "People in twelve-step fellowships have the ability to find recovery from active addiction through working the Twelve Steps."

PRUDENCE
Carefulness, caution, discretion. Good sense, forethought. Responsible behavior, doing what is necessary or warranted, without making rash or frivolous decisions. An individual using discretion with resources, money, or actions is showing prudence.

Related to Traditions Seven and Nine and Concepts Five and Eleven, a group or service body in twelve-step programs is charged with being prudent, or responsible, with fellowship money.

PUBLIC INFORMATION/PUBLIC RELATIONS
Image management, publicity, marketing. The process of making others aware of an organization by various available media, including flyers, mailers, presentations, advertisements, television, radio, movies and the Internet. As related to recovery, offering information about the primary purpose of an organization, where meetings may be found, etc.

The Eleventh Tradition advises that recovery fellowships should only engage in a public relations policy of "attraction rather than promotion."

PUBLIC INFORMATION (PI) SUBCOMMITTEE
A service body or committee found in most twelve-step fellowships that is tasked with informing the public of the existence of the fellowship through the use of various print media, meeting with professionals in the business community, and literature and meeting schedule distribution. Some of these PI subcommittees also manage a phone line/hotline for people to call in to request information about the fellowship. This is terminology specific to the service structure found in most twelve-step fellowships.

Qq

QUALIFICATION

A speech, (called a "pitch" in some twelve-step fellowships) delivered by a member at a recovery meeting. Differs from a "share" at an open or discussion meeting in length and formality. A qualification is often an autobiographical recounting of the member's life experiences before and after he or she entered recovery, and as such is his or her "qualification" for program membership—although no formal qualifications exist. The pitch is generally uplifting, conveying the speaker's "experience, strength, and hope" for the benefit of newcomers and others in attendance.

Also relates to service in twelve-step fellowships wherein members offer their qualifications for a particular service position as a trusted servant.

QUALIFIER

In recovery fellowships such as Nar-Anon, Al-Anon, or Sex and Love Addicts Anonymous—which exist for the recovery of those in relationships with addicts or alcoholics or those for whom relationships themselves are an addiction—a "qualifier" is the person or the relationship to whom the member is addicted.

Rr

RAGE

Temper, wrath, fury. Intense anger, often manifesting itself in violence. A very serious and intense expression of the feeling of anger, which if not addressed or treated, can be damaging to the recovery process and to relationships. Anger is a normal human emotion, but if it gets out of control or out of balance, it can become rage. Acting on rage is usually indicative of more serious issues. Considered a character defect.

RATIONALIZE

Justify, explain, defend. To attempt to make one's behavior or past actions seem reasonable, or try to make unacceptable behavior appear acceptable. People with the disease of addiction often rationalize their addictive behaviors; this is also part of the denial that is present with addiction. Rationalization is considered a character defect.

RCM (REGIONAL COMMITTEE MEMBER)

A program member elected to represent his or her area on the regional service committee (RSC). An area may have two regional committee members. An RCM carries the area conscience on motions on which votes have been cast, learns about upcoming events, and is the link between the area service committee and the regional service committee. This is terminology specific to the service structure found in most twelve-step fellowships.

RD (REGIONAL DELEGATE)

A member elected by the regional service committee to carry the regional conscience to the world service conference. The RD is the link between the regional service conference and the world service conference and traditionally is responsible for conducting service workshops and/or conference agenda workshops. This is terminology specific to the service structure found in most twelve-step fellowships.

READY

Prepared, equipped, organized. The Sixth Step says one must be "entirely ready" to ask a higher power to remove his or her character defects—this means to have no reservations, doubts, or hesitation. To be in a state of willingness and preparedness.

REALITY

Truth, actuality, existence. That which actually could or does exist, as opposed to an imaginary or false nature. The state of being from which drugs and alcohol often provided an escape. In recovery, one embraces reality or "life on life's terms," one does not attempt to escape from it.

REBELLIOUSNESS

Defiance, obstinacy, noncompliance. Rebellion is often the act of doing something simply because it is the opposite of what another person or group wishes one to do. Considered a character defect.

RECIPROCAL

Joint, shared, mutual. Characterized by give-and-take. Describes the action of returning what was given in kind or providing another thing in return that is of equal or greater value. A sponsorship relationship, friendship, or any relationship wherein two people give to one another equally or nearly so. Reciprocity is one of the main components of the Twelfth Step.

RECOVERY

Revival, healing, revitalization. A return to a former state of usefulness or health. As related to recovery from addiction, the process of building a new, drug-free life out of the desperation of active addiction. The process of getting and staying clean/sober/abstinent.

Recovery has a meaning far beyond the idea of mere abstinence, and it includes the process of correcting behaviors or learning new and healthier patterns for one's life through working and living the Twelve Steps. Recovery is a lifelong process with many different mechanisms, systems, or components, but predominately involving the Twelve Steps. To live a life in recovery is to live in freedom from the slavery of addiction and in a full, rich, and rewarding way that has meaning and value. The definition of recovery is evolving and a source of debate in addiction-recovery-treatment communities. Some believe in medication-assisted recovery while others believe in total abstinence.

REGRET

Remorse, grief, repentance. A feeling of sorrow, shame, or guilt about one's past behaviors or events that took place in the past. Having a guilty conscience or feeling shame because of the damage one has caused or the wreckage one has created. To feel unhappy about missing an opportunity or not taking positive advantage of a situation when it presented itself. To feel responsible for the things done when one was in active addiction.

RELAPSE

Setback, deterioration, decline. To "go back to." As related to recovery, the state of returning to an old pattern of behavior, whether it is using alcohol or other drugs or negative, maladaptive behavior that varies according to any number of manifestations of one's addiction.

Relapse is a process that begins when a person stops taking the necessary actions to maintain his or her spiritual fitness (such as going to meetings, staying in contact with a sponsor, being of service, and working the Twelve Steps), and culminates in the actual use of mind- and mood-altering chemicals or the return to a destructive behavior. Relapse does occur; however, it is not a part of the recovery process.

RELATED FACILITIES AND OUTSIDE ENTERPRISES

Excerpt from the Sixth Tradition. This usually refers to treatment centers and/or hospitals that treat individuals with addiction, but may also refer to clubhouses or other structures.

RELATIONSHIP(S)

Association, liaison, bond. A relationship is a connection between ideas, things, or people. Types include intimate, sexual, family, marital, romantic, sponsorship, acquaintance, etc. Establishing and maintaining communication with another individual or group and having shared experiences with each other are generally considered important parts of relationships.

The Twelve Steps teaches members to build and nurture relationships with a higher power of their understanding, others, and themselves.

RELIGION

Creed, faith, belief. The organized study of the divine or spiritual aspect of life. Compliance with a way of life that its advocates believe puts them into a relationship with the divine.

A group or organization devoted to a particular belief system and usually with a single leader, responsible for the group, who is in the position to give directives to the members. A group of people who worship the same idea of a deity in a certain traditional or ritualistic manner.

REMORSE

Regret, guilt, shame. The feeling of responsibility, sadness, or sorrow for past actions. Not to be wallowed-in; however, it is possible that being aware of one's remorse can have a positive effect if it motivates a person to change his or her behavior.

REPARATION(S)

Compensation, reimbursement, damages. As related to the Ninth Step, the action of making amends by taking responsibility for one's actions. May include approaching the person one has harmed, taking responsibility for the incident or situation, and offering to repair the situation in either a financial manner or through action. This includes rectifying a situation when possible and making every effort to live in such a way as will not cause damage or harm in the future.

REPRESSION

Subjugation, suppression, oppression. "Squashing," pushing down feelings or knowledge about unpleasant or painful realities. For some victims of abuse or extreme stress, repression keeps painful memories from conscious awareness; persons in recovery may repress true knowledge of harms they have done (this is not the same as a "blackout," which is an involuntary neurological phenomenon, not a mental one). Repression and suppression are both defense mechanisms; though related, they are distinct from each other.

REPRIEVE

Pardon, acquittal, amnesty. To give temporary relief or delay from punishment or pain. In recovery, it is believed one achieves only a reprieve from active addiction, not a permanent cure. The length and quality of the reprieve depends upon the degree of one's practice of the Twelve Steps.

RESCUE

Save, set free, release. To assist a person to safety or free him or her from danger. In recovery, may be the well-intentioned action of interfering with another person's recovery by preventing him or her from facing the consequences of his or her actions.

RESENTMENT

Grudge, bitterness, to feel offended. Ill feelings for a person, place, or institution with which one has come into conflict. Often these feelings will linger long after the initial problem is resolved. Resentment causes a person to relive a situation repeatedly, instead of attempting to let go or surrender. Even when a person has a legitimate grievance, to hang on to old resentments only damages his or her prospects for recovery. Holding onto a resentment and/or being resentful is considered a character defect.

RESERVATION

Stipulation, reluctance, provision. A loophole left in a recovery program that may lead to a relapse. Considered insidious and often hidden; a person may not realize he or she has any. Examples include: "If my mother, father, child, spouse, etc. dies, I don't know if I can stay in recovery," or, "If I find out I have a deadly disease, I am going to use again."

RESISTANCE

Opposition, refusal, defiance. A negative reaction to trying anything new, such as recovery. The opposite of open-mindedness and willingness, two qualities necessary for recovery.

RESOURCES

Assets, means, source of supply. As related to recovery, something that can offer assistance, such as a sponsor, recovery literature, meeting attendance, reaching out to others, the fellowship, a peer or support group, friends with more time in recovery than one has, service commitments, etc.; anything that an individual can access to assist with the process of recovery.

RESPECT

Esteem, reverence, high regard. A spiritual principle, it includes admiration or deference toward a person or group. Those in recovery should also respect the power of the disease of addiction if they want to stay in the recovery process.

RESPONSIBILITY

Accountability, dependability, conscientiousness. Being able to be relied upon. Doing the work necessary to provide for one's needs. Not relying or depending on another to do work that one can/should do for him- or herself. Making decisions and thinking about how the consequences may affect others.

A spiritual principle embodied in the Twelve Steps, which teaches members to take responsibility for their recovery by seeking solutions to problems that may arise.

RESTITUTION

Recompense, amends, compensation. Part of the Ninth Step amends process. To offer an equivalent of any loss or damage one may have caused during his or her active addiction. However, the Ninth Step cautions "except when to do so would injure them or others."

RESTORATION

Return, restitution, re-establishment. The process of returning something to a previous or former state of health, perfection, or wholeness. The Second Step states that a higher power can "restore" our sanity, indicating that we once enjoyed the state of mental health and can again through the twelve-step process. Also part of the Ninth Step amends process as one seeks to restore relationships that have been damaged by active addiction.

RESULTS

Consequences, outcomes, effects. The evidence of work completed. What a recovering person gets out of working the Twelve Steps that is directly proportionate to the effort he or she puts into the recovery program. A few examples of these results may be building time in recovery, social acceptability, healthy relationships, employment, or spiritual, emotional, mental, and physical balance.

REVEAL

Disclose, tell, make public. To make something visible or uncover something. By continuing to work the program in all aspects of one's life, "more will be revealed" about oneself, one's relationship with one's higher power, and one's relationships with others.

RIGHTEOUSNESS

Virtue, morality, decency. The character trait of doing the right things for the right reasons; behaving in a just or honest manner with integrity and self-respect. Behaving properly can be a result of working a recovery program and learning how to live right. However, *self*-righteousness is often used to prop up one's own ego and make others feel small; it is considered a character defect.

RIGID

Inflexible, unbending, stiff. Not flexible, pliant, or moving. Fixed in idea, attitude, perception, or action. Being rigid in one's beliefs or attitudes is the opposite of open-mindedness and is considered a character defect.

RIGOROUS

Exact, thorough, meticulous. A continuous and regular effort in a particular area; building strength and stamina. Steady effort put into a program of recovery, creating results based on the Twelve Steps that foster great growth.

RISK

Jeopardy, danger, threat. Also refers to the act of taking the chance of losing one thing in order to gain another; maybe losing a negative quality or virtue in order to gain a positive asset. Venturing out of one's comfort zone in order to grow, learn something new, etc.

re·cov·er·y |ri'kəvərē|

Ss

SABOTAGE/SABOTAGING

Damage, disruption, interference. Destruction of property or obstruction of normal operations. Treacherous action to defeat or hinder a current path, cause, or an endeavor. The deliberate or unconscious destruction or derailment of one's life. Those in twelve-step programs often refer to sabotaging their programs by not working the steps, calling their sponsor, or following basic suggestions offered by those with long-term recovery.

SANITY

Mental health, good sense, wisdom. The ability to deal with reality as it is. The state of being sane, rational, or having a sound mind; results in healthy decision-making based on knowledge of real-life experience and consequences rather than on fantasy or wishful thinking. Part of the Second Step in which one can be "restored to sanity" by coming to believe in a higher power.

SARCASM/SARCASTIC

Irony, mockery, scorn. Using words as a weapon against another person, often disguised as humor, but at the expense of another. Can be a form of passive-aggressive behavior toward another. Making exaggerated, false, or overblown statements at odds with reality, e.g., pointing out when someone does something foolish, "Oh, *that* was smart," in order to make the other person feel inadequate would be sarcastic. Considered a character defect.

SEARCHING

Penetrating, probing, incisive. Related to Step Four; a "searching and fearless moral inventory" is a penetrating and honest evaluation of the ways addiction affected every area of one's life, including acknowledgment of addiction's effects on the lives of others. A searching inventory leaves nothing out, and digs deeper than surface level circumstances to discover the root of the problem, issue, or behavior. To discover the motives, desires, or expectations that underlie one's behaviors.

SECOND STEP

From the Twelve Steps (Step Two). It states that a person begins to believe that his or her sanity can be restored by a higher power.

SECOND TRADITION

From the Twelve Traditions (Tradition Two). It states that for purposes of the twelve-step group there are no leaders, but that there is one "ultimate authority, a loving God as he may express himself in the group conscience." Leaders are described as "trusted servants . . . (who) do not govern."

SECRET(S)

Clandestine, undisclosed, hidden. Information a person keeps to him- or herself, either personal or about another person or situation. A secret is not shared with another person and might concern past or present behavior or actions one feels shame about. A secret may constitute a reservation in one's program that can contribute to relapse. Undisclosed information about a person that will keep that person sick, prone to relapse, or unable to change behavior in a certain area.

SECURITY

Safety, refuge, sanctuary. Can also mean a guarantee. A feeling of security is needed in order to feel free and able to communicate or express one's feelings in the confidence that one's privacy will be respected.

SELF

Identity, personality, person. Of and pertaining to needs or wants of the individual person, sometimes to the exclusion of others. Selfishness and self-centeredness have long been considered among the defining character defects of those with addiction.

SELF-ABSORPTION

Narcissism, self-importance, vanity. Completely concerned with self. To think only and mostly of self. When a situation arises the first thought is "how will this affect me?" with little or no regard to the effect the situation will have on others. Considered a character defect.

SELF-ACCEPTANCE

Approval of oneself without reservation. The understanding that one has positive as well as negative qualities. The knowledge that nobody, including oneself, has to be perfect in order to belong in this world. A certainty that one is "good enough."

SELF-CENTERED

Egotistical, self-absorbed, selfish. Believing oneself to be the center of any situation, whether in a negative or a positive way (either "everybody hates me" or "everybody loves me"). Evaluating everything and everyone in terms of their relation and usefulness to the self. Similar to self-obsessed. Considered a character defect.

SELF-DECEPTION (SELF-DELUSION)

Lies, fantasies, etc. "told" to the self. A refusal to accept the truth, usually about one's role in past or present wrongdoings. A refusal to acknowledge the reality of a situation or of one's behaviors. The attempt to manage and control one's addiction by making claims that one can stop at any time or that the behavior is not as bad as it actually is are examples of self-deception. Considered a character defect.

SELF-ESTEEM

Self-worth, confidence, self-respect. The value one places on oneself. Depending on one's opinion of oneself, self-esteem is often characterized as "good" or "bad," "high" or "low." In recovery, self-esteem is boosted by performing service, step work, etc.

SELF-HATRED

Self-loathing, disgust of oneself, extreme dislike of oneself. Intense hostility, degradation, or humiliation of oneself, especially because of feelings of guilt or inferiority. Self-hatred can be extremely detrimental to one's recovery and is often considered a character defect.

SELF-OBSESSION

Incessant thoughts of self, fixation on self. An inability to think of anything other than one's own needs and desires, often at the expense of others, and with little or no regard to how one's actions may affect them. Considered a character defect.

SELF-PITY

The belief that one's own life is more difficult, tragic, or sadder than that of anyone else. This feeling is usually accompanied by a lack of gratitude and makes it difficult to remember that in each life there are both negative and positive elements. Considered a character defect.

SELF-RESPECT

Self-worth, dignity, confidence. The act of honoring one's self in manner, behavior, and/or interaction with others. A habit of reverence for self and for acting with integrity and with regard for the effect one's actions will have on the self and others. Considered a spiritual principle.

SELF-RIGHTEOUS(NESS)

Smug, sanctimonious, pompous. The belief that one is always correct or that one knows more than others. The inability to admit when one is wrong. Often accompanied by attempts to defend one's own actions or point of view at all costs or at the expense of others. May be the result of fear, and is often a way to deflect criticism or make others out to be insignificant. Considered a character defect.

SELF-SEEKING

Egocentric, egotistical, vain. Always looking for ways to attract attention or to improve one's own position at the cost of others. This characteristic may cause one to try to become a "big shot" or "guru" in his or her fellowship, boasting of the number of sponsees he or she has, the speed with which he or she did the steps, etc. Considered a character defect.

SELF-SUFFICIENT (SELF-SUFFICIENCY)

Autonomous, self-contained, independent. Usually a positive trait, but may be considered unhealthy when it prevents someone in recovery from establishing a relationship with or accepting help from his or her higher power or others in recovery. May be related to a lack of trust or faith.

SELF-SUPPORTING

Self-financing, successful, self-sustaining. All twelve-step fellowships follow the Seventh Tradition injunction to be "self-supporting through our own contributions." This is to avoid the problems of outside influence (interference) that accepting donations from those outside the fellowships would inevitably involve.

SELF-WILL

Stubbornness, willfulness, obstinacy. Often viewed as a negative in twelve-step fellowships. Determination to have one's own way. Generally seen as contrary to the will of one's higher power.

However, when regarded philosophically, everything a person does voluntarily, whether healthy or unhealthy, reflects self-will in action.

SELF-WORTH

Self-respect, self-esteem, confidence. The value one places on him-
or herself. Generally, one's self-worth is low after a period of active
addiction. Living in recovery almost always results in an elevated sense
of self-worth.

SELFISH

Egotistical, greedy, self-centered. Believing or acting as if one's wants
or needs are of greater importance than the wants or needs of another.
Thinking only of oneself and putting the rights, wants, needs, or desires
of others second. Considered a character defect.

SENSITIVE

Perceptive, susceptible, receptive. Easily hurt or upset; touchy. Inversely,
can mean alert, finely tuned, responsive.

Persons in active addiction often demonstrate extreme sensitivity to
slights (real or perceived) against themselves, but not so much to the
feelings of others. The twelve-step process enables people in recovery to
turn that sensitivity outward, and instead of focusing on their own hurt
feelings, respond to the hurts felt by others and try to help them.

SERENITY

Peacefulness, tranquility, contentment. A sense of calm during crisis,
stress, complications, and upsets. Serenity is the hallmark of recovery—
rather than feeling the old edginess, restlessness, and impatience of
addictive needs that can never really be satisfied.

Serenity means feeling grounded and connected to one's higher power
and to the people who surround one; feeling connected to one's life, and
being physically, mentally, emotionally, and spiritually balanced. Serenity
can be achieved through prayer and meditation and when practicing the
Twelve Steps.

SERVICE

Aid, assistance, benefaction. Helping other people, groups, or institutions; usually associated with volunteering one's time and committing a certain portion of that time either once or on a regular basis. In a meeting, service may consist of setting up, cleaning up, sharing when called upon, making coffee, or serving as a group's secretary, treasurer, or chairperson. Sponsorship or area-, regional-, or world-level commitments are forms of service, as is contributing during the Seventh-Step collection.

SERVICE BOARDS

As defined in the Ninth Tradition, service boards can be created in order to serve the fellowship. These boards consist of members elected by a service committee and are "directly responsible to those they serve." Many twelve-step fellowships have service boards to oversee an office or corporate entity, such as a district or central office of a twelve-step fellowship, as well as various workgroups focused on developing literature and other needs as outlined by the fellowship. This is terminology specific to the service structure found in most twelve-step fellowships.

SERVICE CENTERS

A physical structure/building that is usually a literature distribution center, meeting facility for service boards, information clearinghouse, and more. Funded through a combination of member, area, and regional donations, as well as by literature sales. Service centers may employ program members to do jobs that would ordinarily have to be done by nonmembers, which is not the same as paying a recovering person for service work. Service work is done as a part of working the Twelfth Step and is strictly unpaid. People who work at service centers are typically called special workers. The concept of employing special workers at service centers is addressed in Tradition Eight. This is terminology specific to the service structure found in most twelve-step fellowships.

SEVENTH STEP

From the Twelve Steps (Step Seven). It requires one to humbly ask his or her higher power to remove his or her shortcomings (character defects). Step Seven begins with the word "humbly," which indicates that humility is the key to this step. Humility is distinctly different from humiliation; it is a realistic acceptance of one's own humanity—one's assets as well as deficiencies—and involves the knowledge that help is needed in order to continue on the path of recovery.

SEVENTH TRADITION

From the Twelve Traditions (Tradition Seven). It states that each twelve-step group should support itself financially and not accept funding or donations from outside organizations or nonmembers. This is to avoid the problems of outside influence (interference) that accepting donations from those outside the fellowships would inevitably involve, discussed in the section on self-sufficiency, above. Being self-supporting is also a way of being responsible for oneself at the group level.

SEX ADDICTS ANONYMOUS (SAA)

A twelve-step fellowship of men and women who admit their powerlessness over addictive sexual behavior. The goal of the SAA program is abstinence from one or more specific sexual behaviors; however, unlike other programs, Sex Addicts Anonymous does not have a universal definition of abstinence. Rather, the members seek to abstain from both obsessive mental preoccupation with sex and compulsive sexual behavior. SAA was founded in 1977 and has meetings in more than twenty-four countries, including the US. The recovery text for SAA is called *Sex Addicts Anonymous*, also known as the SAA Green Book.

SEXAHOLICS ANONYMOUS (SA)

A twelve-step fellowship for individuals who have a desire to stop lusting and become sexually sober. The primary purpose of SA is to stay sexually sober and help others to achieve sexual sobriety. Lust is considered to be the reason why SA members act out sexually. Sexual sobriety is achieved when members do not act out on lust. SA was founded in the late 1970s by Roy K and has a service office located in Tennessee. *Sexaholics Anonymous* is the fellowship's recovery text. There are SA meetings in the US and forty-seven countries worldwide.

SEX AND LOVE ADDICTS ANONYMOUS (SLAA)

A twelve-step fellowship of men and women whose primary focus is to help each other recover from sex and love addiction. Members believe that this addiction may take several different forms including, but not limited to, a compulsive need for sex, extreme dependency on one or many people, or a chronic preoccupation with romance, intrigue, or fantasy. Its recovery text is called *Sex and Love Addicts Anonymous*. There are SLAA meetings in twenty-five countries, including the US.

SEXUAL COMPULSIVES ANONYMOUS (SCA)

A twelve-step fellowship of men and women whose primary purpose is to recover from sexual compulsion and stay sexually sober. Members are encouraged to develop their own definition of sexual sobriety as well as their own sexual recovery plan. SCA started in 1973 and has a recovery text called *Sexual Compulsives Anonymous: A Program of Recovery*, also known as The Little Blue Book.

SHAME

Disgrace, dishonor, humiliation. A painful feeling many persons continue to carry into recovery. Shame involves regret or embarrassment because of immoral, dangerous, illegal, etc. past activities either engaged in to obtain and use substances or act on addictive behavior, or due to the lack of inhibition produced by active addiction. Shame can be addressed and relieved by completing thorough Fourth and Fifth Steps, as well as after Ninth Step amends are made.

SHARE (SHARING)

Impart, reveal, disclose. Speaking up when called on in a twelve-step meeting for the purpose of letting members of the group know more about the speaker's "experience, strength, and hope." This allows newcomers in the group to learn how the program works and what it has done for others, familiarizes newcomers with potential sponsors, and contributes to the feeling of fellowship within the group. Each group and meeting has different guidelines and etiquette for sharing.

SHORTCOMINGS

Inadequacies, failings, faults. Related to the character defects that were revealed in the Fourth and Fifth Steps, and which the Seventh Step seeks to have one's higher power remove.

SIGNIFICANT OTHER

Life partner, mate, companion. May be a spouse or live-in lover. Not reflective of any specific sexual orientation or lifestyle.

SIMPLE

Uncomplicated, straightforward, easy. Desirable in recovery, reflected in such expressions as "keep it simple." Twelve-step fellowships often refer to themselves as "simple programs for complicated people."

SIXTH STEP

From the Twelve Steps (Step Six). The basis of this step is for the recovering person to become completely willing to have his or her character defects removed.

SIXTH TRADITION

From the Twelve Traditions (Tradition Six). States that twelve-step groups should never endorse any related businesses or institutions in case problems, such as ownership, status, or finance, divert the group from its original goal of helping persons seeking recovery.

SNIPER SHARING

Contradicting or criticizing a previous speaker while sharing at a twelve-step meeting. When sharing, it is customary to share one's "experience, strength, and hope." Opinions do vary and a person may disagree with what someone else has shared in a respectful manner without "sniping," or making obvious or pointed remarks or insults.

If a member has a problem with another member's sharing, it should be discussed person-to-person, respectfully, after the meeting.

SOBER

Alcoholics who are in recovery refer to themselves as "sober" members of their fellowship. In sex addition recovery, being "sober" refers to abstaining from romantic or sexual behaviors one has identified as troublesome. These are classified, during work with one's SA, SAA, or SLAA sponsor, as "inner circle" or "bottom line" behaviors—behaviors one has agreed not to engage in at risk of having a relapse.

SOBRIETY

Abstinence, clear-headedness, temperance. Terminology used primarily in the fellowship of Alcoholics Anonymous. The state of being free from the drug alcohol.

"Sobriety" is considered in a similar vein as "recovery," as a state of being that is very desirable, positive, and enriching, a way of life that includes adherence to twelve-step principles, and that is much more than mere "abstinence" or "being dry."

Used in sex addiction recovery, the word "sobriety" describes the state that a person recovering from sex, lust, love, and/or a relationship addiction is in while working his or her program. This person would be abstaining from bottom line or inner-circle behaviors, attending meetings, not engaging in enmeshed relationships, or acting out in any number of other sexual behaviors.

SOCIALLY ACCEPTABLE/SOCIAL ACCEPTABILITY

Not stigmatized, not demonized. Something regarded as tolerable and respectable by the public. Relating to the manner in which people in groups behave and interact with one another, "socially acceptable" refers to what is considered "good" behavior, cooperation, kindness, etc.

Something that is socially acceptable is considered either a benign or a positive influence on the community, causing no harm to others.

SOLUTION(S)

Answer, explanation, resolution. The key to a puzzle or the answer to a problem. In recovery, the Twelve Steps are pointed out as a solution to the disease of addiction.

SPECIAL INTEREST MEETING

Sometimes called "common needs" meetings. The primary purpose of these meetings is always to carry the message of recovery to the person who suffers from addiction. No person in recovery will be turned away even if they do not belong to the common need or special interest group (a referral may be made to a general interest group after the meeting). Examples of special interest meetings may include meetings for young people; gay, lesbian, bisexual, and transgendered (GLBT) people; women only; men only; professionals (e.g., doctors, lawyers, entertainers, etc.) for whom anonymity may be especially important or difficult to achieve in an ordinary open or closed twelve-step meeting.

SPECIAL WORKERS

Individuals, whether in recovery or not, who are employed by and paid for their work at service centers/offices for twelve-step programs/ fellowships. Referenced in Tradition Eight.

SPIRIT

Courage, strength, force. The unseen quality within a human being that is not physical; that which motivates an individual to evolve or connect to a higher power or from which the feelings of an individual stem. That part of the being connected to a higher consciousness. Sometimes called soul, essence, inner self, life-force, and/or chi.

SPIRITUAL

Sacred, holy, transcendent. Of or pertaining to the non-material, non-physical. The belief in a higher power, higher consciousness, or universal truths; not necessarily a "God" associated with religion. Having to do with principles that are timeless and universal instead of immediate and particular. Having a focus on a collective well-being as opposed to only being concerned with the self.

SPIRITUAL AWAKENING

An awareness of one's own authentic nature. Having insight into one's life that was previously unavailable. Transcending a current situation and viewing that situation with a different opinion, feeling, or perception. The realization that one has the ability to live by principles.

The Twelfth Step says that once one has had a spiritual awakening as the result of working the Twelve Steps, the next action is to carry the message to those who still suffer (from any manifestation of the disease of addiction) who wish to recover.

SPIRITUAL PRINCIPLES

Philosophy, values, beliefs. As related to the spiritual principles found within the steps, these are a suggested code of conduct by which to live. Positive actions, sometimes called "opposite actions," that recovering people strive to live by and are found embodied in the Twelve Steps, Twelve Traditions, and Twelve Concepts. Examples include: hope, faith, trust, patience, courage, perseverance, humility, honesty, willingness, open-mindedness, service, anonymity, tolerance, compassion, etc.

SPIRITUALITY

Belief in or practice of transcending the human experience of survival and meeting carnal needs in pursuit of something higher, be it a higher consciousness or higher power. The pursuit of connection with a universal truth or consciousness. The act of striving for transcendence of a current situation in pursuit of a higher, deeper, wiser understanding and/or connectedness.

SPONSOR

Supporter, liaison, backer. A person who guides another person through working the Twelve Steps. A sponsor need not have any particular length of recovery, but it is generally thought that he or she should have a sponsor of his or her own, should have worked the Twelve Steps him- or herself, and participate in his or her chosen fellowship. It is suggested that every recovering person acquire and use the assistance of a sponsor when working the Twelve Steps.

SPONSORSHIP

The relationship between two recovering people wherein one serves as a mentor, teacher, or guide through the Twelve Steps of the program. The act of sponsoring another person. Sponsors each have their own ways of working with their sponsees. There is no one way to sponsor.

SPONSORSHIP FAMILY

A group of recovering persons connected through sponsorship. A "grand-sponsor" is the person who sponsors the sponsor; "great grand-sponsor" sponsors the grand-sponsor; "sponsee brothers" or "sponsee sisters" share the same sponsor. These are not official titles, simply affectionate terms that have become accepted through usage over time. These people may also become part of the recovering person's support group. Some coordinate gatherings, weekend events, or private meetings to celebrate their recovery together as "families."

STAYING CLEAN

Remaining spotless, fresh, unspoiled. To continue to be abstinent from all mind- and mood-altering chemicals and activities with the purpose of recovering from addiction to them. Substances and activities may include alcohol and/or other drugs, compulsive gambling, sex, shopping, video gaming, etc.

STEP EIGHT

From the Twelve Steps (Eighth Step). Requires the recovering individual to make a list of the people he or she has harmed and be willing to make amends to them all. The Fourth Step inventory is usually used as a resource to help develop the Eighth Step list, as, paradoxically, often it is the people one has harmed whom one resents, and their names are typically on the Fourth Step list of wrongdoings and resentments.

STEP ELEVEN

From the Twelve Steps (Eleventh Step). Calls for prayer and meditation to improve conscious contact with one's higher power. According to the step, one's prayer should only be to gain knowledge of that higher power's will and the ability to carry it out.

STEP FIVE

From the Twelve Steps (Fifth Step). It calls for those in recovery to admit to their higher power, another person, and to themselves the exact nature of their wrongs. The step during which an individual in recovery relates the inventory created during the Fourth Step to his or her sponsor or other trusted person, and discusses the findings thereof with a focus to become willing to remove the defects revealed in the inventory.

STEP FOUR

From the Twelve Steps (Fourth Step). The person in recovery is instructed to perform a "searching and fearless" moral inventory. The methods of working this step may vary according to fellowship attended. For example, some fellowships have people write a narrative/story or make a list or write in columns, but whatever format is followed, the Fourth Step inventory is a written assessment by a person in recovery of his or her own past deeds, revealing resentments, strengths and weaknesses, character defects, and all aspects of his or her relationships, assets as well as defects. The point is to "inventory" one's character and to get rid of what is damaged and to examine what needs to be built up for continued healthy growth.

The Fourth Step is often approached with great fear by the newcomer, but there is no need for this. All the millions of people, all over the world, who have attained lasting, long-term recovery through twelve-step programs, have taken Fourth Steps. While writing down one's past deeds might be embarrassing or even emotionally upsetting, it is never going to be as bad as having done those deeds in the first place. An understanding sponsor will be of great help in taking this step.

Old timers who have gone through the steps, including the Fourth Step, numerous times, insist that the Fourth Step is where true relief from the suffering of addiction begins.

STEP NINE

From the Twelve Steps (Ninth Step). It calls for the recovering person to make amends to all people he or she has harmed (listed in Step Eight), except when doing so would cause further harm to either the injured party or others.

STEP ONE

From the Twelve Steps (First Step). Requires the acknowledgment of powerlessness over one's addiction, coupled with an admission that one's life has become unmanageable. It is often said in twelve-step fellowships that this is the only step that must be done to perfection, as it logically calls for abstinence, which is the prerequisite for recovery. The admission of powerlessness paves the way for a realistic opinion of the self and lays the foundation for all the other steps.

STEP SEVEN

From the Twelve Steps (Seventh Step). Requires that the recovering person asks his or her higher power to remove his or her shortcomings in a spirit of humility. This may be done through formal prayer or though a simple, conversational request to the God of one's own understanding.

STEP SIX

From the Twelve Steps (Sixth Step). States that the recovering person has become entirely willing to have his or her higher power remove his or her character defects.

STEP TEN

From the Twelve Steps (Tenth Step). Requires ongoing personal inventories and continued admission of any wrongdoing, as soon as possible after it is recognized.

STEP THREE

From the Twelve Steps (Third Step). The recovering person is directed to make a decision to turn his or her will over to a higher power as that person understands that power.

STEP TWELVE

From the Twelve Steps (Twelfth Step). It states that after completion of the steps and having a spiritual awakening because of working those steps, the person in recovery must now try to carry the message of recovery to other people suffering from addiction and practice the spiritual principles in all of his or her affairs.

STEP TWO

From the Twelve Steps (Second Step). It declares that a person has come to believe that a power greater than him- or herself could restore him or her to sanity.

STEP ZERO

Humorous reference to all the everyday living that many addicts must relearn or learn for the first time. Learning to perform the daily "basics" of life prior to working a First Step; consists of things such as getting regular rest, making one's bed, eating three meals a day, attending to personal hygiene and health, daily meeting attendance, learning to pray, doing laundry, learning to make phone calls to friends in recovery, reading recovery literature, etc.

These things were typically neglected in active addiction, so relearning them or learning to do them for the first time lays the groundwork for doing the Twelve Steps and participating in the recovery fellowship of one's choice.

STEPS (TWELVE STEPS)

The Twelve Steps are the basis of all recovery programs referred to as "twelve-step programs." Originally developed by the founders of Alcoholics Anonymous and based on the "Four Absolutes" of the Oxford Group (an early Christian-based group with an interest in helping alcoholics or drunkards, as they were then called). Because the steps work when one works them, the Twelve Steps have become the "gold standard" for treating every manifestation of addiction, from overeating to pornography.

The Twelve Steps are worked in a specific order because each one lays the foundation for the next. This sequential process assists a person in recovering from addiction. The steps are best done under a sponsor's guidance. There is no timetable for completing the steps.

STRENGTH

Potency, vigor, might. The power or perseverance necessary to complete a task or cope with a situation or issue.

SUBSTITUTION

Switch, exchange, swap. Replacing one object, thing, or behavior with another. The act of putting down one behavior or substance to pick up another or allowing the disease of addiction to manifest itself in different ways.

SUCCESS

Victory, triumph, achievement. An accomplishment. Success for a person in recovery might not consist of material wealth, but may simply be living serenely without picking up, relapsing, or acting out one day at a time.

SUGGESTIONS

Proposals, propositions, ideas. Recommendations based on the successes and failures of others who have attempted the same task and learned what works and what does not work. Not carrying the weight of commands or laws, suggestions may simply be concepts that have been successful for other members of recovery in collective experience.

SUICIDE

Deliberate self-killing; intentional, self-inflicted death. Suicide occurs in every culture, all over the world, in every age group and social class. Addiction increases the risk of deliberate suicide, as well as the risk of accidental self-killing by overdose. Active addiction is often considered to be a form of gradual suicide.

Also refers to the concept of doing something that may be against one's own best interests leading to loss of reputation, financial loss, etc.

SUPPORT

Carry, sustain, maintain. To offer assistance to someone. Listening to someone who needs to talk, taking someone to a meeting, or staying after a meeting to talk with someone are all examples of support in recovery.

SUPPORT GROUP

Support groups typically have members who share common experiences and/or circumstances and can empathize with each other. It is a place where people can give and receive emotional, medical, spiritual, or other useful support, as well as exchange information. In addition to twelve-step support groups, there are groups for people living with grief and loss, those living with chronic pain or illness, specific groups for any number of medical conditions, groups dedicated to a spiritual or religious sect, etc.

A group of clean/sober/abstinent people who assist one another in the recovery process. A support group may engage in service or social activities together. Central to this group will usually be a sponsor, sponsorship-family members, and those with whom one regularly attends meetings.

SURRENDER

Submit, yield, capitulate. To lay down arms, stop fighting, concede. Recovery begins with surrender, an admission of powerlessness—whether conscious or not—that whatever the individual was clinging to must be abandoned, whether it was alcohol, other drugs, or a behavior. Once that initial surrender or "giving up" takes place, others follow, until the person realizes that "giving up" or surrendering to the will of the higher power is, in fact, the way to "win" a new and healthy life.

SURVIVE

Endure, live on, continue to exist. Also to last longer than, or live through, especially relating to a challenge or crisis.

SYMPTOMS

Warning signs, indications, evidence of an illness. Symptoms of the disease of addiction go beyond the substance or behavior to which one is addicted. Examples of some of these symptoms, in addition to the more overt physical symptoms, include: progression of use of substances and/ or destructive behaviors, obsession, loss of control, compulsive use, and continuing to use despite negative consequences.

Tt

TAPES

Recordings, messages; from the technology of audio- or videotape, the recorded sounds or images of words or scenes. Used to refer to the succession of thoughts or ideas that stream through a person's mind when he or she contemplates addictive or other negative, damaging behaviors.

"Playing the tape out" is another way of saying "thinking an idea through to the end," noting all the possible consequences and ramifications.

"Playing old tapes" may also refer to listening to old (mental) messages that tell one that he or she will never succeed in recovery, is "too old, too fat, too stupid, etc." to become a person in recovery. Listening to these old, negative messages may lead to relapse.

TEACHABLE

Capable of being instructed; having the ability to listen to and benefit from lessons, examples, advice; to remain willing to learn and have an open mind. To know that there is always more to learn. To be open to continuing growth. Being teachable is an important quality in recovery.

TEMPTATION

Attraction, inducement, lure. As related to recovery, a situation or "trigger" that creates an overwhelming idea or thought of using or acting out on one's addiction. Anything that produces an extreme desire to use or act on one's addiction.

TENTH STEP

From the Twelve Steps (Step Ten). It calls for continuing to take a personal inventory and when wrong, promptly admitting it.

TENTH TRADITION

From the Twelve Traditions (Tradition Ten). States that twelve-step programs have no opinion on outside issues so that the program's name and/or reputation are never drawn into public controversy.

THANKFUL

Gratified, appreciative, pleased. The state of being grateful for what one has or is given or what one has always had, but never before appreciated. A necessary state for ongoing recovery. Considered a spiritual principle.

THERAPEUTIC

Restorative, healing, beneficial. Leading to health. Can refer to behavior or the attempt to treat or cure a disease, illness, or injury.

THIRD STEP

From the Twelve Steps (Step Three). It requires making a decision to turn one's will over to a higher power as one understands that power.

THIRD TRADITION

From the Twelve Traditions (Tradition Three). A guiding principle stating that the only requirement for membership in a twelve-step program is the desire to stop either using, drinking, or acting on an addictive behavior. As long as one has this desire, no one else, in or out of the fellowship, can deny one membership or meeting attendance.

THIRD STEP PRAYER

A prayer many in recovery say, privately, throughout the day, or aloud and in unison at meetings. The exact wording of the prayer varies depending on the twelve-step program, but comes from the Third Step of those programs and involves asking a higher power to guide one's will and life, and guide one in his or her recovery; thereby showing one how to live by the principles of the program.

THIRTEENTH-STEPPING/THIRTEENTH STEP

A somewhat glib euphemism for what occurs when a member with a greater amount of time in recovery dates (or attempts to date) someone with less time in recovery, i.e., a newcomer. Considered predatory and dangerous, especially to the newcomer, who needs time and space to get his or her bearings, come to grips with newly uncovered emotions, and is usually in great pain and need. Given this volatile mix of conditions, a newcomer is often "ripe for the picking" by those who should know better. Known Thirteenth-Steppers are not accorded respect in twelve-step programs. Those who engage in this type of behavior can be male or female, straight, gay, or bisexual. Thirteenth-stepping in recovery fellowships can be compared to sexual harassment in the workplace.

THOROUGH

Meticulous, methodical, systematic. To follow through to completion. As related to recovery, to be complete, searching, and leave nothing undisclosed. The Fourth Step calls for a thorough moral inventory; leaving nothing out.

TOLERANCE

Open-mindedness, broadmindedness, acceptance of the differing views of other people. "Live and let live" is an expression of tolerance. Neither tolerance nor acceptance should be confused with approval. Considered a spiritual principle.

TOOLS

Apparatus, utensils, gear. In recovery, "tools" refer to the actions, prior experiences, or spiritual principles that can assist a recovering person to get and stay in recovery. Examples include: having and using a sponsor, belonging to and phoning a support group, attending twelve-step meetings, reading recovery literature, having and keeping a service commitment, journaling, and working the Twelve Steps. Tools may be acquired from listening and sharing in meetings about what has worked for other recovering people and from active participation in the program.

TRADITIONS (TWELVE TRADITIONS)

Twelve guiding principles for the twelve-step groups that help to ensure the program continues and thrives. Originally written soon after the establishment of Alcoholics Anonymous, and adapted by other twelve-step programs, the Twelve Traditions apply to the fellowship in the same way the steps apply to the individual in recovery. The traditions provide a structure and outline the way in which the groups should relate to their members, the members to the groups, and the way the fellowship itself should relate to the world at large.

TRIGGERS

Prompts, instigators, stimuli. Sense memories, situations, or people from an individual's past that begin the thought process of using or engaging in maladaptive behaviors. Anything that provokes the desire to use.

A trigger is anything that sets off a compulsion or urge within a recovering person that may result in his or her getting loaded or acting out on addictive behavior. Triggers may include people, places, or things, such as bars, songs, smells, driving through certain neighborhoods, or seeing certain people whom the individual associates with old behaviors, having cash in one's pocket or wallet, getting angry, getting a pleasant surprise, payday, etc.

TRUST

Confidence, reliance, belief. An important component in recovery and key to developing a relationship with a higher power. Trust is necessary between sponsor and sponsee, and often develops between the recovering person and the group. Considered a spiritual principle.

TRUSTWORTHY

Dependable, reliable, honest. A trustworthy person may be relied upon to keep promises and live up to responsibilities. A person in recovery learns that the way to gain others' trust is by being trustworthy. Considered a spiritual principle.

TWELFTH STEP

From the Twelve Steps (Step Twelve). It states that once a person has had a spiritual awakening as a result of working the first eleven steps, he or she must carry the message of recovery to others suffering from addiction and to practice the spiritual principles of the program in all of his or her affairs.

TWELFTH TRADITION

From the Twelve Traditions (Tradition Twelve). States that anonymity is the foundation of all of the Twelve Traditions and advises placing principles before personalities. The emphasis on principles rather than on individual personalities is intended to promote true humility based on an understanding that all are equal in the twelve-step fellowship, that there are no "big shots," and that the only true authority comes from one's higher power.

Uu

ULTIMATE AUTHORITY

The final, definitive, greatest, or supreme power, one without equal.
In twelve-step recovery, refers to the higher power, which many equate
with the idea of God. In the Second Tradition, reference to the "ultimate
authority" is framed by the idea that twelve-step fellowships have no one
person who "manages" or "directs" others; rather there is one "ultimate
authority," a "loving God" as expressed in the "group conscience" of
fellowship members. Twelve-step-fellowship leaders are simply "trusted
servants; they do not govern."

UNCONDITIONAL LOVE

Affection and positive regard given freely, without boundaries,
requirements, or reservations. Loving someone "no matter what." Does
not mean tolerating any unacceptable behavior, it means that love
will never be withdrawn on the basis of some action by the loved one.
Considered a spiritual principle.

UNDERSTANDING

Sympathetic, comprehension, insight. Understanding others helps one be
patient, tolerant, and accepting of them. Considered a spiritual principle.

UNFORGIVING

Intolerant, callous, vindictive. Reluctant or refusing to forgive. Providing little or no opportunity to forestall undesired results or mistakes. Considered a character defect.

UNIFORMITY

Sameness, consistency, standardization. Following a set order, pattern, plan, etc. Although twelve-step fellowships emphasize unity and common purpose as the way to recovery, unity is not the same as uniformity. The rooms of twelve-step fellowships are filled with diverse groups of individuals who would ordinarily not get together, all trying to solve a common problem.

UNIQUE

One-of-a-kind, distinctive, rare. Something different or special from other things; out-of-the-ordinary. People in recovery (especially those new to the process) often feel unique, but not in a good way; they may feel themselves exempt from the workings and traditions of the twelve-step group or of life itself because of some special status, or they may feel unique in their isolation, or they may feel such shame and guilt over their past deeds that they are sure they are unique in all the world in their wrongdoings. Whatever the reason, feeling unique may be deadly for a recovering person. The phrase "terminal uniqueness" was coined to emphasize just how deadly feeling unique can be for a person trying to recover from addiction.

UNITY

Harmony, accord, unison. The state of being unified or united; being part of a cohesive group. In twelve-step terms, "unity of purpose" keeps the groups focused on the core problem the members are gathered to address. Referenced in Tradition One, ". . . personal recovery depends on NA (AA/GA/OA/SAA/etc.) unity."

UNIVERSAL

Collective, total, entire. Having application to everyone, everywhere at all times. Spiritual principles are universal, and apply to everyone, everywhere, whether one realizes this or not.

UNMANAGEABILITY

Unruliness, disorderliness, unable to be controlled, regulated, or ordered. Unmanageability may express itself in the life of a person suffering with addiction as job and marriage problems, arrests and incarcerations, serious debts, inability to pay bills, the inability to form and nurture relationships, etc. Considered a character defect.

UNREALISTIC EXPECTATIONS

Wants or desires regarding an outcome from a person, group, or particular situation that are not viable, that cannot happen, or that would not be healthy if they came to pass. Placing demands or conditions on a person or situation that cannot be met; setting the stage for disappointment or resentment, which can be deadly for persons in recovery.

UNWILLINGNESS

Recalcitrance, disinclination, obstinacy. Reluctance to perform an action or take a step. Considered a character defect.

USELESSNESS

Ineffectiveness, inutility, inadequacy. Without purpose. Individuals still in active addiction often report feeling hopeless, that their lives are meaningless, or without any direction; they describe themselves as lost, confused, or depressed in active addiction. Living a life in recovery and especially being of service to others restores a feeling of usefulness to the life of a recovering person.

USER

Consumer, customer, abuser. In twelve-step programs, user relates to those who use mind- and mood-altering chemicals and/or engage in maladaptive, addictive behaviors. Can also refer to people who take advantage of other people or who are manipulative, using others to achieve their own ends. Similar to being a "taker" rather than a "giver."

USING

The act of taking into the body mind- and mood-altering chemicals or engaging in behavior to which one is addicted. The act of fixating on a person, place, activity, or thing in order to fill a void inside the addicted individual that could otherwise be filled with the principles of recovery.

USING DREAMS/DRUNK DREAMS

Dreams in which the dreamer experiences the sensations of being high, loaded or drunk, or engaging in addictive behavior. Settings may include old behaviors associated with using. They are not predictive of relapse or indicative of a deficiency in the dreamer's program of recovery, such as a reservation.

re·cov·er·y |riˈkəvərē|

Vv

VALUES

Principles, standards, morals. Also refers to ethics or ideals. Values may belong to a person or a group. Value can also mean "worth." A person in recovery gives great worth to the concept of honesty; it is a value for that person.

VENGEFUL

Resentful, unforgiving, ruthless. Desiring vengeance or being vindictive. Proceeding from a desire for revenge or serving to exact vengeance. Considered a character defect.

VICES

Immoral behaviors, bad habits, faults. Addiction itself is not a vice; it is a disease. Vices, however, may be manifestations of the disease of addiction. Vices are considered character defects.

VIGILANCE

Attention, watchfulness, alertness. To be constantly and continually aware of situations, feelings, and behaviors that pose dangers to one's spiritual condition. Continuously working on recovery: praying, meditating, regularly attending meetings, etc. Self-monitoring to ensure adherence to one's program of recovery.

VIOLENCE

Brutality, cruelty, hostility. Any act of physical, emotional, verbal aggression, or hostility. Considered a character defect.

VULNERABLE

Susceptible, defenseless, weak. May be a feeling of being unprotected or at risk. Sharing or revealing intimate details about oneself with others may lead to feelings of vulnerability. Allowing oneself to be open or transparent to another; putting oneself in a situation that could result in having one's behaviors or actions called into question. Paradoxically, when people in recovery attempt to hide or deny their vulnerabilities, instead of strengthening their recovery, they often become more prone to relapse. By making oneself vulnerable, that is, by sharing one's thoughts and feelings with others in recovery, one often finds strength.

re·cov·er·y |ri'kəvərē|

Ww

WE

The Twelve Steps of Narcotics Anonymous, adapted from the Twelve Steps of Alcoholics Anonymous, added the word "We" to the beginning of Steps Two through Eleven, in order to emphasize that recovery is a "we" endeavor, not a solitary or isolated activity to be engaged in alone.

WELCOME

To greet or receive. Used as a salutation for newcomers and out-of-town visitors who identify themselves as such at meetings.

WILLINGNESS

Eagerness, enthusiasm, readiness. A key character asset said to be all that is required of a newcomer or old timer in working the program. The desire to complete a task and the decision to do whatever is necessary to accomplish it. Willingness gives one the ability to take action, to attend meetings, work steps, do service work, get and use a sponsor, and especially to be open-minded. Considered a spiritual principle.

WILLPOWER

Determination, resolve, drive. Self-control or self-discipline. No matter how much a person suffering with addiction tries to stop using on willpower alone, he or she is usually unsuccessful without a program of recovery.

WINNER

Victor, champion, conqueror. One who does not give in to difficulties, but perseveres and continues to act upon spiritual principles, no matter who else is involved in the situation. People who do not use alcohol or other drugs or act on an addictive behavior. Winners are people who go to meetings regularly, work the Twelve Steps with a sponsor, volunteer for service work, help newcomers, and participate in other healthy, positive activities. Winners are those who strive to exemplify the characteristics of a healthy recovering person.

WISDOM

Knowledge, insight, astuteness. May be learned or gained from one's own past personal experiences or by observing and learning from the collective experiences of others.

WITHDRAWAL

As related to addiction recovery, the physical, emotional, and psychological reactions the body experiences in the absence of a particular substance or combination of substances (detoxification). Takes place whether the substances used were prescribed or illicit (illegal/street) drugs, medications, food, alcohol, or behavioral addictions such as sex, overeating, or gambling.

Symptoms may include, but are not limited to: vomiting, nausea, aches, pains, seizures, headaches, sweats, flu-like symptoms, depression, anxiety, difficulty focusing, etc. Individuals may require hospitalization during the beginning, detoxification phase of withdrawal. This decision can be made by a medical doctor.

Withdrawal lasts varying amounts of time, depending on types of drugs or behavior, combinations of drugs used, length of usage, length of relationship, health of the individual, and other factors.

Withdrawal generally occurs at the very beginning of recovery; only when all intoxicating substances and behaviors have been removed can the recovery process begin in earnest. Emotional withdrawal symptoms may last longer, but gradually subside just as the physical symptoms do.

WORKAHOLICS ANONYMOUS (WA)

Workaholics Anonymous is a twelve-step fellowship of individuals whose primary focus is to help each other to stop working compulsively. The WA definition of abstinence is "to abstain from compulsive working, activity, worry, and work avoidance." The fellowship began in New York in 1983 and has a primary recovery text titled *The Workaholics Anonymous Book of Recovery*. There are meetings worldwide, including the US.

WORRY

Anxiety, stress, fear. Discomfort or unease. Mental distress related to a given or feared outcome. Worry should be avoided by persons in recovery as much as possible. Sharing concerns with a sponsor is one way to drain worries of their power. Sharing at group level or with recovery friends is also helpful.

WORTH

Importance, value, meaning. The merit or significance of a thing; be it concrete or abstract. One's recovery is worth any amount of time or effort. Self-worth may be identified through working steps and identifying one's character assets.

WORTHWHILE

Important, meaningful, valuable. Deserving of the time and effort spent on it, like one's recovery.

WORTHY

Admirable, commendable, praiseworthy. The quality or state of being deserving. Persons newly in recovery may feel they are not worthy of the love and friendship of other members of the fellowship, but after some time, and especially while living by the principles of the Twelve Steps and performing commendable actions such as being of service, one usually begins to realize one is worthy of recovery.

WRITING PROCESS

The method of working the Twelve Steps by answering questions about them, writing one's thoughts about and understandings of them in one's journal or notebook, done under the guidance of a sponsor. The act of listing and describing feelings, thoughts, ideas, etc. on paper and then reading what one has written to a sponsor or another guide through the Twelve Steps. Writing is an important part of twelve-step recovery.

WRONGS (WRONGDOINGS)

Crimes, injuries, wounds. The hurtful and/or injurious things one has done to others; what others have suffered because of one's active addiction. These are the things the Ninth-Step amends process is designed to address.

re·cov·er·y |ri'kəvərē|

Zz

ZEAL

Passion, enthusiasm, gusto. Excitement and eagerness for something—
a cause, a belief, a way of life, etc. The feeling one has for one's
program of recovery, which causes one to embrace the twelve-step
way of life enthusiastically.

ZEALOT

Fanatic, enthusiast, believer. A person who is extremely committed
to a cause or belief. Can also refer to someone who is overly adherent
to a religious sect. While it is not necessarily a negative for those
new to the recovery process to be zealots, it is best to strive to live a
recovery-oriented life with balance and moderation.

re·cov·er·y |ri'kəvərē|

FAQs and General Program Facts

The following are some of the more common questions and more detailed answers about attending meetings. There are many more questions and far more answers than space permits, but this is intended as a good start (and good refresher) for people attending a meeting of any twelve-step program.

How do I identify/What do I say?

You've almost certainly heard the formula, in movies or on TV: "Hello, my name is X, and I'm a Y." If you are attending a meeting for the first time, pay attention to what other people are saying and try to emulate them. As a general rule, you do not need to identify as "something and something," for example as "an addict *and* an alcoholic," regardless of whether you are attending Alcoholics Anonymous or Narcotics Anonymous. If you are still deciding if you are suffering from addiction, you don't have to identify as anything. Simply stating your first name is sufficient.

Naturally, there are varying opinions on this subject, but generally speaking, if you are attending an NA meeting, you should say "addict" and identify your amount of time in the program as "clean time" or "recovery." If you are attending AA, you should say "alcoholic" and identify your amount of time in the program as "sobriety."

Where do I sit?

It is best to sit in a place where you will not be distracted and can focus on those who are sharing. Some meetings will fill up from front-to-back, while others will fill back-to-front. Many meetings in urban or densely populated areas are standing-room-only after a certain time, so get to the meeting early and get a seat. It is generally accepted to save a couple of seats until the meeting fills up. If people are standing or looking for seats close to the start time, common courtesy says you should give up the saved seat(s). Remember, getting to a meeting early enough to get a seat is the responsibility of the program member; he or she will understand why you could not hold a seat indefinitely.

Can I go outside during the meeting?

If you need to use the restroom or wish to smoke, just exit the meeting quietly. If you need to leave the meeting early, simply gather your things and, if absolutely necessary, quietly excuse yourself to your immediate neighbors.

What if I am late?

There's a saying—"the only meeting you're ever late for is your first one." Of course, it's best to arrive early, but many programs believe it is better to arrive late to a meeting than not at all. In smaller meetings it may be more noticeable if you arrive late, but it is completely normal and accepted to come in to a meeting late. Just remember that a meeting *is* going on and try not to be distracting. Many recovery veterans believe in getting to the meeting place early for the informal "meeting before the meeting," and staying to socialize or "fellowship" after the meeting ends, for "the meeting after the meeting."

How long do I need to stay in the meeting?

The general rule is, "prayer to prayer." If you really want the full benefit of the meeting experience, then you should stay from the opening prayer to the closing prayer. Most people in recovery will also say, "Get there early and stay late." Much of what happens in recovery takes place before and after the meeting, during the informal period of "fellowshipping." It's the best way for people to get to know you and for you get to know other recovering people.

What are milestones of recovery?

Typically, milestones of recovery in twelve-step programs are at thirty, sixty, and ninety days; six and nine months (and in some fellowships, eighteen months); and every 365 days in recovery thereafter—in some parts of the country they are called anniversaries, and in other parts birthdays. Milestones are usually acknowledged at a meeting, either weekly or monthly, in a variety of different ways, according to local and fellowship custom.

What about meeting attendance or court cards?

If you have an attendance or court card requiring a signature, place it in the basket that is passed for the Seventh Tradition. Usually the meeting secretary or treasurer will sign it and then make it available to you after the meeting has ended. This is done as a courtesy to you; the group is not required to sign your card. Please wait until the end of the meeting to get your card back. And never interrupt the meeting by trying to get a meeting attendance card signed for a meeting that you intend to leave early.

What if I want to go to a meeting to "check things out" for myself or a friend? What if I'm not quite sure that I have a problem?

Find an open meeting. Most meetings will be described in program schedules as either "open" or "closed." Schedules are also available online in most areas. If you call a central office or hotline number, ask the person who answers the phone to guide you. A meeting that is listed as open is considered open to anyone who wants to attend. These open meetings are usually where family members or friends attend with their loved ones who are in recovery. Open meetings are where people who are unsure if they have a problem can find more information to help them make an informed decision.

Do I have to stop: using, drinking, gambling, spending, shopping, smoking, having sex, being compulsive or codependent, etc. before I can attend a meeting?

No, but it *is* strongly suggested that you do not bring with you any drugs, paraphernalia, or any items considered a threat to the members of the fellowship you are attending; however, if you do show up to a meeting loaded or drunk, no one will ask you to leave unless you are also belligerent or seem extremely ill. Remember, the people in the meeting may be in recovery now, but they have experience being around those who are still in active addiction. You will not frighten them or make them want to use. You are not that powerful.

Are there managers or bosses at groups or meetings?

No, but most meetings do have a secretary or chairperson and other volunteers who set up the room, hand out group readings, and/or find speakers for the meeting. These fellowship members (referred to in program literature as "trusted servants") are not serving in any official or corporate capacity; rather, they are elected by other group members and are willing to serve the group. All service positions in twelve-step programs are voluntary, and members serve on a rotating schedule.

What is the difference between meetings and groups?

A group can be defined as two or more persons who come together for the specific purpose of sharing their recovery from whatever manifestation their addiction takes with other persons also seeking recovery. Meetings are basically gatherings that usually take place at regularly scheduled times and locations. A group may hold a number of meetings, e.g., on different days of the week. A meeting may include newcomers, old timers, out-of-town visitors, and "regulars" or members who have been attending the same meeting together for some time.

A group essentially organizes a meeting; a group usually has a name and adheres to an agreed-upon format (speaker, book study, open discussion, etc.). Groups are generally considered the foundation for the service structure of most twelve-step fellowships. Meetings may coalesce around a common theme or membership feature; hence, there may be gay groups, women's groups, men's stag groups, "old timers" groups, young people's groups, and so on.

What is a home group?

Persons seeking recovery are welcome to attend any meeting of whichever fellowship addresses their particular problem. However, most people find it important to "belong" to one particular group, which they call their "home group." Some fellowships strongly recommend home group membership and service.

In the home group, the recovering person finds friendship and fellowship and may accept service responsibilities. Home group members attend business meetings of the group, organize special events for the group, and help set up and clean up after meetings. The home group is often simply the group within which the recovering person feels most comfortable; sometimes a home group is chosen because it is the group a person's sponsor belongs to.

Typical service positions in a home group include secretary or chairperson, treasurer, group representative, coffee person, literature person, greeter, and other positions. The secretary or chairperson is usually responsible for selecting members who will then lead the meeting; a secretary may make announcements, share, open and close the meeting, and make sure other service positions are fulfilled.

There also are elected positions filled by members of the group. These group positions are known as the group service representative (GSR) and the alternate group service representative. Typically, groups will hold a "business meeting" or "steering meeting" once a month. At these meetings, any monies collected by the group over and above what is needed for rent and coffee, are banked or otherwise earmarked by group conscience to make a contribution to the next level of service, such as a central office or area service committee.

GSRs carry the conscience of the group to the area service committee meeting, which is usually held once a month.

Sharing and introductions.

At the beginning of some meetings (usually closed meetings and not often in very large meetings) everyone in the room will take turns to introduce themselves. Other than that, it is always common practice for the person who shares to introduce him- or herself by saying his or her first name and identifying in the way that is accepted by that group or program, as in, *"My name is Jane, and I am an [addict, alcoholic, compulsive gambler, etc.]."* In most cases, you do not need to identify with more than one manifestation of addiction. It is redundant and unnecessary to say "addict and alcoholic" for example. Alcoholics are, by definition, addicts. If you are at an AA meeting, the reason for your attendance is to address your addiction to alcohol and not other drugs. Similarly, if you are in a meeting of NA, you only need identify as an addict.

If you are asked to identify yourself at your first meeting and are not yet comfortable with that identification, you can simply say your name and that you are not sure you have a problem and that you came to the meeting to learn more. You will be welcome to stay either way.

At some meetings, group members will also acknowledge their recovery date or the date on which their recovery began, such as, "My name is John and I'm an addict with four years clean." This, however, is usually more common in newcomer groups or therapeutic groups that are not twelve-step oriented.

Sharing.

You (usually) will only be asked to share at a meeting if you have been abstinent for at least twenty-four hours. Don't be offended if you are not asked to share at your first meeting; the members may have noted your nervousness as a newcomer (after all, each of them was in your seat, once), and they may be respecting your need to "feel better" before they ask you to share.

Some meetings run on the "tag" system, with each person who shares "tagging" or selecting the next member to share. Until you have attended a few of these meetings, and the other members get to know your name, they may not call on you. A newcomer may not be called on for another reason; the program members may wish to hear about recovery, and until you have some recovery time under your belt, you can't say very much about that subject.

Often newcomers will share about events in their past that took place while they were still in active addiction, since that is basically all they have to share. These "drugalogs" or "drunkalogs," while certainly not forbidden, take the focus off recovery, and talking about addiction, substance abuse, or the ways in which you acted prior to recovery just isn't that interesting to most individuals in recovery. Old timers have a saying, "What the newcomer's got, we got rid of. We want to hear about the solution, not the problem."

Listen to the sharing of others and observe how long they speak (or if the meeting has a suggested time limit, respect it). Do the same when it is your turn to share. Twelve-step groups are not therapy sessions. Any advice or commentary you wish to make regarding something you hear shared in a meeting is best addressed privately after the meeting.

No cross-talk.

"Cross-talk" is the practice of speaking directly to a person who has shared at a meeting and/or offering advice or commentary to them after their share. This is another way that twelve-step meetings differ from group therapy. Cross-talk is never acceptable. In some areas, checking emails or texting is considered the equivalent of cross-talk, because it prevents at least one person in the room—the one using the device—from listening to the message of recovery. It also distracts others, who may need to hear what is being discussed.

Members attempting to share their personal stories honestly before the group do not need the commentary, advice, or jokes of others present. If people were permitted to remark on each other's sharing, the meeting could very easily become sidetracked, and the primary purpose—recovery—forgotten.

Members usually enjoy each other's company and even tease each other, call each other nicknames, and refer to what was shared, but during the meeting such joking is very limited and the atmosphere returns to the business of recovery quickly. Recovery is not punishment for having the disease of addiction, it is the process of getting better—and there is much laughter in the rooms, as fellowship members realize how much they have in common. This atmosphere of fun is perfectly acceptable and even encouraged. But recovery is also a matter of life and death, and most persons in recovery meetings do take their recovery, but not themselves, seriously.

It is never appropriate to make abusive, racist, sexist, or homophobic comments, or to share in such crude ways as to offend others in the room. If you do so you may not be asked to share again in that group.

Your sponsor or program friends will undoubtedly let you know if your sharing was inappropriate; more often, other members may approach you after the meeting to compliment you on what you shared. Either way, it usually is done in the spirit of helping and fellowship.

Starting a group or meeting.

Before you start a meeting, some thought should be given to the following:

- the need for a meeting in your area/vicinity;
- approval or support from your area service committee;
- intended meeting location and associated costs, and
- prospective attendees—those in recovery who can help support the meeting as it gets off the ground.

Most area service committees in the various twelve-step fellowships have a literature distribution subcommittee and often help new meetings by providing a group starter kit that contains information pamphlets, group readings, and/or key tags, as well as helpful information about starting a meeting or group.

Prayers at meetings.

Most twelve-step meetings usually will open and close with a prayer (you may show respect by standing silently if you don't wish to join in). These prayers are not intended to promote any particular sect or denomination of any particular faith, though some of them may sound familiar to you. The "Lord's Prayer" is commonly heard at AA meetings, while at NA and GA meetings it is generally not. Some prayers will have the word "God" in them, but this is meant as the God of one's own understanding and not meant to denote a specific denomination. Twelve-step recovery is spiritual in nature, not religious.

Atmosphere of recovery.

Each meeting can be as different as the members who attend it. Some meetings are more social, standing-room-only types of meetings, while others are more serious, intimate, or quiet. Some meetings are somber and focused, while others may be more genial and comradely. Whatever the type of meeting, an atmosphere of recovery is established and maintained by a few rules. These generally include a ban on the overt use of cell phones or other communication devices (even in a silent mode, for texting), dissuasion against private conversations during sharing, and a request that all in attendance respect the needs of the group. Remember, members are dealing with life-and-death issues, and some of the newer attendees may be emotionally fragile and need to be able to hear what the speakers are sharing. Since twelve-step programs operate on a basis of "attraction, not promotion," boorish, unruly, or rude behavior might prove a turnoff to someone who sorely needs the program, but who is repelled by what he or she perceives as the values of the group.

The norms of the group will usually become evident over time, whether lenient or strict. Also contributing to the atmosphere of recovery is respect for the meeting facility and acknowledgement that the actions of any particular group do reflect on the twelve-step program as a whole. One disrespectful group may spoil a meeting location for other groups.

Disturbances at meetings.

Attendance at many twelve-step meetings is open to the public. This enables newcomers to investigate the program before making a decision to join. However, it also means that on occasion, a person who is still under the influence or suffering from a mental disorder other than addiction finds his or her way into a twelve-step meeting. Opinions are divided as to the best way to deal with such persons; however, the group conscience must make a final determination on a case-by-case basis (unless there is an immediate danger).

People with mental or emotional difficulties are often able to benefit from attendance, and if they are able to conform to meeting etiquette, nothing further need be said or done. If a person is overly emotional, disruptive, or seems violent, the more experienced group members are usually able to assess and handle the situation. A business meeting may need to be called to address the situation if it persists.

The guiding principle should be: No one who seeks recovery should ever be unwelcome at a twelve-step meeting, but conversely, no one should feel unduly uncomfortable or threatened in a meeting.

Special Interest or Common Needs meetings.

Most twelve-step programs have meetings that are specifically targeted at certain populations. These may be established for men only, women only, gay, lesbian, bisexual, and transgender (GLBT) only, young people only, or professionals. Each type of meeting calls for special notice of its own membership and practices. A few examples of special interest or common needs meetings are:

- **Stag (Men's or Women's) meetings**

  "Stag" (gender-specific) groups provide an opportunity for men to share about feelings and behaviors they would feel awkward discussing in front of women, and vice-versa. These meetings also provide opportunities for women to find women sponsors and men to do likewise with men. Much bonding and fellowshipping is possible in these same-sex meetings (sometimes called "buddying-up"). If you find yourself in a meeting for the opposite gender, don't be offended if you are redirected to another meeting; on the other hand, you may be invited to stay, for that one meeting at least.

- **GLBT meetings**

  GLBT meetings originated in part as a result of the AIDS epidemic; in the early years of the crisis, many, if not most of those infected with the virus were gay, and of course those gay addicts and alcoholics wanted to share at meetings about this terrible disease and its impact on their lives. There's still debate as to whether it was fear of the disease or plain bigotry that led heterosexual program members to insist that sharing about AIDS was an "outside issue," but whatever the reason, GLBT addicts and alcoholics branched out and formed their own groups where they could discuss their special fears and concerns as well as their recovery.

Now research has proven that many behaviors—not only those associated with homosexual activity, but also some associated with addiction—dispose a person to contract the virus that causes AIDS (and many addicts have learned that behaviors they engaged in might be responsible for their contracting Hepatitis C). AIDS is known to have been contracted through sharing needles, blood transfusions or other medical procedures, and in varied other ways, and is no longer considered a "gay disease"; its sufferers in recovery no longer have a double stigma. But the GLBT affinity groups that sprouted as a result of the AIDS epidemic have proven to be valued by many gay, lesbian, bisexual, and transgendered people in recovery, and they flourish today.

• Young People's meetings

There is not a clear definition of how old a "young" person should be, but as more facts become known about addiction, people are no longer waiting until middle age to enter recovery; it's not uncommon for teenagers to have multiple years in a program. An acceptable age for a "young person" at a meeting so specified would be from about mid-teens to late twenties.

• Professional meetings

In some twelve-step fellowships, there may be certain meetings not on any official schedule. These undisclosed meetings may be for professionals such as doctors, lawyers, politicians, nurses, and/or celebrities whose livelihood depends on an even greater degree of anonymity than that practiced in regular twelve-step meetings.

Meeting formats.

Even within the various fellowships, there are different formats for twelve-step meetings. The names and descriptions will vary depending on geographic locations, local customs, and the differences in twelve-step programs. The descriptions below offer a general overview. Meeting directories and Internet sites usually will have a legend to direct you to the meeting type you want to attend.

Open meetings are open to anyone who wants to attend, including family, friends, or members of the public who are simply interested in getting more information about the program.

Closed meetings are only for people who are members of the program or who have the desire to stop using or acting on their addiction.

Newcomer meetings focus on specific issues that are common to those who are new to the twelve-step program and the recovery process. Some issues discussed may include finding a sponsor, establishing a meeting habit, or the first three steps.

Speaker meetings feature one or more members who share their experiences by telling the story of what active addiction was like, what early recovery was like, and what their life is like now. These shares vary in length depending on the meeting and may last anywhere from fifteen to forty-five minutes, sometimes followed by question-and-answer or open participation from others in attendance at the meeting.

Step (or Tradition) Study meetings as the name suggests, focus on a specific step or tradition at each meeting. Text regarding the step or tradition being studied is usually read aloud from approved program literature, the leader or chairperson discusses his or her interpretation or experience with that step, and sharing may or may not follow, which could include a question-and-answer session.

Discussion or Open Participation meetings have a leader or chairperson who starts the meeting off with a general share of a few minutes, then selects a topic, and then either calls on people to share or acknowledges volunteers who wish to speak. Sharing happens in a variety of ways at any given meeting, including the raising of hands, calling out at the end of another's share, "tag" meetings where at the end of his or her sharing, the speaker calls on the next person (sometimes called Monterey-style sharing), and so on. The format of the meeting will usually be announced at the beginning. Some meetings appoint members who act as timers to make sure that one person does not dominate/monopolize the sharing so that all who wish to may participate.

Book Study meetings refer to reading the program's literature, including, but not limited to, its primary text and additional conference-approved literature.

Candlelight meetings are those with muted lighting that is thought to make it easier for some people to share and also contributes to an atmosphere of calm and serenity.

Getting "kicked out" of a meeting.

You cannot get "kicked out" of a twelve-step program. You can, however, be asked to leave a particular meeting place or location because your behavior is disruptive or you are not following group or facility rules. If you are asked to leave a meeting location by the secretary or elected representative of the group you are obligated to leave that space. A law enforcement official could be called in, and a charge of trespassing pressed. This is an extreme situation, but may be necessary, and if so, is well within the legal rights of a group and its trusted servants.

re·cov·er·y |ri'kəvərē|

Meeting and Fellowship Etiquette

Going to one's first meeting of any twelve-step program can be a nerve-wracking, confusing, and for some, frightening experience. A person attending a meeting for the first time can take comfort in knowing that *each and every person* at the meeting had to go through the same experience of walking into that room for the first time. Every member or potential member faced the fear of identifying him- or herself as an addict, alcoholic, overeater, compulsive gambler, codependent, sex and love addict, etc. and then taking that first key tag or chip. Regardless of the length of recovery, there was a time when every single person at that meeting had only one day. That is, perhaps, the most important thing to remember.

"Meeting and Fellowship Etiquette" is intended as an easy guide to help you understand what to expect when you walk through the door of your first meeting, and what to do while you're there. We hope this guide will be useful for both newcomer and old timer alike. Showing respect for each group, listening to the members of that group, and following the meeting format will help any newcomer (or old timer) have a positive and uplifting meeting experience.

What is meeting etiquette?

Meeting etiquette consists of customs, manners, and propriety; it is the way to conduct oneself while in a recovery meeting. Meeting and fellowship etiquette has become an important topic among many members of the twelve-step community, as well as those who refer people to the various twelve-step programs. People "associated," but not "affiliated" with twelve-step recovery, such as judges, law enforcement and medical professionals, and others are taking an increasing interest in what actually happens to a newcomer being sent to his or her first meeting. These professionals want to ensure that any newcomer is treated with respect and that those people they refer to meetings are not taken advantage of. They also want to ensure that the meetings actually provide those services as presented in the public relations material from various twelve-step service bodies.

Meeting etiquette has traditionally been a concept passed down from one recovering person to another, e.g., from sponsor to sponsee or a more experienced member to the newer member. There is no standard or accepted model beyond what is written in the Twelve Traditions; however, it is common for each member to take personal responsibility for his or her own fellowship and to make certain that there is an atmosphere of recovery found in the meetings. Most "violations" of meeting etiquette are usually addressed by more long-standing members of a group, usually in a kind and tolerant way.

Examples of meeting etiquette are as follows:

- ◆ Getting to a meeting early enables an attendee to get a beverage, use the restroom, socialize, etc., so they can:
  - › Be sure of a seat before the meeting begins;
  - › Avoid the disruption of performing these activities while members are reading or sharing.

- ◆ Leaving and returning to one's seat or speaking to one's neighbors during the meeting is frowned upon, as this distracts those who may be sharing or those attempting to pay attention.

- ◆ If asked to read one of the passages or literature selections, it is considered respectful to read it as written, without adding comments or "sound effects." The literature of each twelve-step program was written with great care to be of help to those who suffer with addiction. It was voted on by group conscience and each fellowship as a body agreed on the final presentation. Anyone with a disagreement on a particular reading should simply excuse him- or herself from reading it aloud and discuss it afterward, privately, with a sponsor or other program member. "Editorial comments" or "callbacks" in a meeting might confuse or alarm newcomers or others who desperately need to hear the message of recovery as it was intended.

- Using only the language and literature consistent with the twelve-step meeting you are attending ensures that a clear message of recovery is being offered. Using mixed language from various fellowships sends mixed messages and can cause newer members to be confused about the meeting's primary purpose.

- The guideline against "cross-talking" or "sniper sharing" (see page 209) helps maintain a calm and safe atmosphere of recovery in the meetings.

- "Stay in the meeting *'from prayer to prayer.'*" Since most meetings begin and end with a prayer, "staying in the meeting from prayer to prayer" means both physical attendance and mental focus on the meeting from beginning to end.

- The Seventh Tradition states that groups should be fully self-supporting and decline outside contributions. This allows twelve-step groups to carry the message the way it was intended, without the influence of outside people or organizations. It is customary to put a contribution in the basket if one can afford to, but it is not required, nor it is appropriate for a visitor (or newcomer in the first thirty days of recovery, in some fellowships).

- Members do not publicly mention specific facilities, treatment centers, detoxification units, hospitals, halfway houses, etc. Doing so is considered an implied endorsement of these facilities/entities by the member. This is especially important if a member serves on an area or regional public information service body. As such, the member is viewed by the public as a representative of his or her fellowship and listeners will think that the fellowship, rather than the member, is endorsing a specific entity.

- Members refer to the meeting by its name rather than the facility where it is held. Referring to a facility may imply a relationship with the facility.

- Members refrain from mentioning specific drugs or tell overly detailed "war stories" ("drunkalogues" or "drugalogues"); it can make others in the meeting uncomfortable if specific drugs or excessive details are mentioned.

- Many groups will ask members to keep their sharing between three to five minutes in order to give everyone who wishes to share a chance to do so. This is especially important if the meeting has a large number of members in attendance.

- Members show respect for the facility where the meeting is held. Twelve-step programs may not be affiliated with the facility, but they have a responsibility to make certain that the meeting area is left in as good a condition or better than it was found. Smokers should dispose of cigarette butts in an appropriate manner, using cigarette receptacles or ashtrays. Be mindful of behavior outside the meeting as well; negative complaints from neighbors to the facility are a direct reflection on the twelve-step group and have caused many groups to lose a meeting place. Many meetings are held in public places. Groups want to make sure that the behavior of a few members does not negatively affect the fellowship as a whole. This is related to the Fourth Tradition that states "Each group should be autonomous except in matters affecting other groups or (insert fellowship here) as a whole."

If someone is being disrespectful or placing the meeting location in jeopardy, then it is usually the responsibility of the chairperson or secretary to bring the issue to that person's attention. However, no person has the power or authority to berate, reprimand, or expel another from a twelve-step program. They can ask an individual not to return to a particular group or facility if chronic negative behavior puts the facility or its members at risk. The meeting secretary has a responsibility to approach the disruptive person and explain, in a respectful manner, why or why not a certain practice is unacceptable.

re·cov·er·y |ri'kəvərē|

re·cov·er·y |riˈkəvərē|

Slogans of Recovery

Introduction

"Easy Does It," "Ninety in Ninety," "Suit up and Show up," "Focus on the Message, not the Messenger"—these and other slogans abound in twelve-step programs and meetings. Each meeting is different and there are tremendous differences in format or style in different geographic areas. Some of the slogans and phrases are fairly common regardless of where someone may attend a meeting, while others are only heard in a handful of programs or certain select cities, states, or countries. Sometimes these slogans or mottos are printed up in fancy type, framed, and hung on the walls of meeting rooms. A newcomer often feels confused, overwhelmed, or even disdainful on encountering these seemingly simple-minded slogans. So what do they all mean?

That's what this introduction aims to explain.

This section on "Slogans of Recovery" is by no means a complete or comprehensive list, but it should provide a reference or starting point for understanding these shorthand messages from twelve-step experience. Use these slogans as you would anything else you hear in a meeting; talk to a more experienced member about them, ask about them, and in the end, come up with a meaning that works for you and disregard what doesn't. Your understanding is sure to grow deeper as you immerse yourself in your chosen fellowship and work the Twelve Steps.

> **A meeting a day keeps the detox away.** Those who attend meetings regularly tend to have a higher success rate than those who do not. Newcomers are encouraged to attend a meeting a day for at least the first ninety days of their recovery, and although there is no mandated minimum number of meetings for newcomers or old timers, frequent meeting attendance contributes to long-term recovery.

> **A new way of life.** "The Twelve Steps have shown me a new way of life." This phrase is often heard at twelve-step meetings and is really just a different way of living the same life, but performing different actions, and having different perceptions, even while living in the same home, family, or job situation. The person in recovery changes, even if all the circumstances of his or her life do not.

> **Act "as if."** A suggestion made to newcomers, implying that if the program seems confusing or odd, to act as others in the program do, until it makes sense—be of service, go to meetings, read recovery literature, etc. Based on the idea that acting happy actually increases one's level of happiness, and that healthy habits are formed by repetition.

> **Addiction is an equal-opportunity destroyer.** Addiction does not discriminate—anyone can be an addict—the teacher, the dentist, the bricklayer, the legislator, the celebrity, etc. Male, female or transgendered, gay or straight, religious or non-religious, rich or poor—addiction is a brain disease with a genetic component. It is not a moral failing. It just exists. Fortunately, so does recovery.

> **An addict alone is in bad company.** The essence of twelve-step programs is experienced when one person in recovery talks to or works with another, whether one-on-one or in a group. Many people in recovery find it easier to talk with someone who has personal experience with addressing the feelings and other manifestations of addiction rather than talking with a professional, such as a therapist, psychiatrist, or clerical person. But because people tended to isolate while in active addiction, it can be difficult for them, once in recovery, to seek the company and counsel of others in the program. This slogan reminds them that it's important to do so. When someone in recovery is alone,

old thoughts and feelings can surface, along with the conviction that getting loaded might be a good idea.

> **Anger is fear in a party dress.** In the recovery community it is generally accepted that the basis of most anger is fear. Addressing the root fear usually gets to the root of the anger.

> **Atmosphere of recovery.** The physical and emotional environment of the twelve-step meeting should be such that it promotes recovery, security, welcome, and acceptance in order to engender hope, especially for newcomers. An atmosphere of recovery is warm, friendly, and takes into account the fear that newcomers or those returning from relapse might be experiencing.

> **Belly-button birthday.** In some parts of the US, recovery milestones are referred to as "anniversaries," while in others it's customary to call them "birthdays." In order to distinguish natal (or biological) birthdays from recovery milestones, they are referred to as "belly-button birthdays."

> **Building a foundation.** Learning the basics of the program, from frequent meeting attendance, to getting a sponsor, to using the phone, to reading program literature, to beginning to work the steps is all part of building a foundation in recovery. On that foundation the member will be able to build a new life. The fundamentals of the program are said to give members the tools to face problems associated with normal, everyday routines that used to seem too challenging or difficult.

> **By the grace of God/There, but for the grace of God, (go I).** These sayings are frequently heard and sound confusingly alike. Both are based in a traditional Judeo-Christian theology; members who are atheist, agnostic, new-age, or followers of Eastern philosophies might instead believe (for example) that personal responsibility is the deciding factor between relapse and recovery.

The first saying, "By the grace of God," indicates that the speaker believes that he or she did not actually cause his or her own good fortune (such as his or her recovery), but that whatever good came to him or her was a freely given gift, or *grace*, from the God of his or her understanding or his or her higher power.

The second, "There, but for the grace of God, (go I)," is frequently used when discussing the misfortune of another. One member's relapse might be cause for concern among the other members of the group who might refer to it in a meeting, not as a matter of gossip, but as a troubling event they are trying to process. In doing so, a clean/sober/abstinent member might remark, "there, but for the grace of God, go I," indicating that he or she credits his or her higher power with keeping him or her clean/ sober/abstinent, coupled with the realization that anyone, including him- or herself, can also relapse. No one is immune.

› **Call your sponsor.** Pick up the telephone and ask for help working the Twelve Steps. A person to whom this is said might be showing signs of being in denial or acting out in some way and may be in need of having another's perspective, particularly that of his or her sponsor.

› **Carry the message; or Carry the message, not the mess.** From the Twelfth Step, the "message" referred to is that of recovery: that any individual can stop using/drinking/acting out/etc. by embracing and practicing the principles embodied in the Twelve Steps and, by doing so, start to enjoy a life free of addiction. This refers to a member's being an example in action, as well as in words, for others seeking recovery. It also refers to sharing, either personally or at a group level, about one's life and recovery experiences.

The second slogan refers to "enabling" others in recovery by being too generous with loans, free rent, free meals, etc. Everyone can use a little help in early recovery, but there is a point at which a helping hand becomes a detriment to the newcomer, preventing him or her from becoming responsible for his or her own recovery.

› **Cash-register honesty.** Honesty in deed as well as in word; when given too much change, a person with "cash-register honesty" promptly calls the mistake to the cashier's attention and returns it, instead of pocketing it. Practicing cash-register honesty is part of working a good program.

› **Change (or Recovery) is a process, not an event.** Most people
with the disease of addiction seem to be more interested in instant
gratification rather than in long-term investments of time and effort
that will bear fruit some time in the future. This saying is intended to
remind them that recovery is a life-long process that will bring benefits
as long as the recovering person makes the efforts recommended by
the program. The point is that one doesn't simply discontinue a certain
behavior and, then "presto," achieves recovery.

Recovery can be thought of as a bank account of sorts that a recovering
person invests in each time he or she goes to a meeting, works the
steps, calls his or her sponsor, meditates, prays, works with a newcomer,
answers the phone when another person in need calls, or stays in
recovery for another day. This bank account is something the person
may access in times of need, when issues come up, or when he or she
has a bad day. Those in recovery never know when they will need to
draw on that reserve; but when that day comes, there must be assets in
the account.

› **Courage to change.** Popular Al-Anon slogan referencing the second
request of the Serenity Prayer that asks for "the courage to change the
things I can." Al-Anon teaches codependents to detach from their
addict or alcoholic with love, and change the only thing they can
change: their self. (Also the title of a popular daily meditation book
used by Al-Anon members.)

› **Cultivate an attitude of gratitude.** Most people in active addiction
have spent their lives looking for more, more, more. In recovery,
serenity can be achieved by being happy with what one has, instead of
always wanting more.

› **Don't quit five minutes before the miracle happens.** It's often the
case that a person in recovery becomes discouraged and wants to give
up right before a breakthrough or solution to a problem occurs (the
"miracle"). Those around that person, who have more time in recovery,
often recognize that this is about to happen and counsels the sufferer
not to give up with these words.

A person in recovery may stop working the program, claiming discouragement, in order to avoid doing some of the hard work of recovery. A sponsor or program friend who understands this and uses this quote might be just the encouragement a person needs to break through to the next level of recovery.

> **Easy does it.** Advice for working every component of a twelve-step program. Since most people in recovery are often "extremists," it's not uncommon for them to want to suddenly master every aspect of their newfound program and fellowship, including their own lives. This is a recipe for disaster. Old timers know that the best way to approach any problem is a bit at a time, not all at once. It is a formula that in many ways defies reason that even the founders of Alcoholics Anonymous did not fully understand. The only thing that is known for sure is that the steps work as they are written. When asked how the steps really work, AA co-founder Bill W said once in an interview, "Slowly."

> **Enjoy life; this is not a dress rehearsal.** Living in the moment or living just for today is the goal of recovery. Learning to appreciate the daily experience rather than dwelling in the past or projecting into the future is considered the key to freedom and peace of mind. Happiness, joy, and serenity are only possible in the present.

> **Experience is what you get when you don't get what you want.** A response to a member who believes his or her prayer wasn't answered. If the desired outcome was not "delivered," then the person who prayed has the opportunity to learn some lessons, including how to cope with disappointment and remain in recovery.

> **Fake it 'til you make it.** Makes the point with humor that in early recovery so much is strange and different that a newcomer is often well advised to simply imitate those in the fellowship who have quality recovery and just do the things those people do until the newcomer understands the program for him- or herself. Note that the slogan says "'til you make it," indicating that the newcomer must eventually "make it" sincerely.

> **First things first.** Often in early recovery, a newcomer begins to look around and become overwhelmed with the desire to "take care of" all the things he or she had neglected during active addiction. For example, unemployment may make it seem like getting a job is the first thing that needs to be done in recovery. Broken relationships may make it seem like reconciliation should be a priority. However, this slogan simplifies matters by reminding those in recovery that the first thing they need to focus on *is* recovery; once that is underway and a relationship with a higher power established, the next things to be taken care of will not only become clear, the way to take care of those things will also be easier.

> **Focus on the message, not the messenger.** It is really easy at a meeting (especially after attending regularly for an extended period of time) to focus on the person who is sharing rather than what the person is sharing. So this saying encourages one to listen to what is being said, rather than judging the person saying it. Time and time again, the most unlikely person delivers the most important message.

> **Focus on the similarities and not the differences;** or **Identify, don't compare.** Denial has killed many people seeking recovery—the feeling that one is different prevents many from accepting the help of a twelve-step program and allows continued using or acting out. Once an individual accepts that he or she has more similarities to, than differences from, other program members, recovery can begin.

> **Friend of Bill.** A member of Alcoholics Anonymous. In order to maintain anonymity or avoid giving offense, upon meeting someone for the first time, a member of AA might ask "Are you a friend of Bill?" If the person is an AA member, he or she will recognize the meaning of the question and can answer yes; if not, no harm has been done. (The "Bill" being referred to is Bill Wilson, who, with Dr. Bob Smith, is credited with founding AA.)

› **Getting back to the basics.** The basics are the fundamentals of twelve-step programs, which include obtaining, calling, and using a sponsor; working the Twelve Steps with that sponsor; attending meetings regularly; fulfilling some sort of service commitment at a group level; and reaching out to others in the program through sharing, calling, or listening to others in recovery. When a recovering person drifts or gets complacent, he or she may have stopped doing the basics of recovery. This often happens because that person has family, school, or work obligations of his or her "new life" and forgets to do the simple things that made that new life possible in the first place. When people in recovery get too far from doing the basics necessary to maintain recovery, they may not be prepared when "life on life's terms" presents itself. Either they will have enough of a foundation to get back to working the program the way they should, or they may relapse.

› **Getting better doesn't always feel better.** The process of working the Twelve Steps, admitting powerlessness, opening one's mind, taking an inventory, looking at character defects, making amends, taking regular personal inventory, engaging in prayer and meditation, and trying to help others—all of these activities are very challenging and may cause disturbances in the familiar cycle of one's own life and thinking, while restructuring one's life and priorities. This restructuring often causes pain or discomfort, as does working out at a gym, for example. "No pain, no gain," is another way to express this concept.

› **The gift of despair/gift of desperation.** The experience of "hitting bottom," with its inescapable shame, degradation, pain, and loss is, in retrospect, often viewed by those in recovery as having been a gift, in that it was the thing that finally stopped them and brought them into recovery.

› **GOD equals Good Orderly Direction.** As early as Step Two, people in recovery are confronted with the need to believe that something (a power) greater than themselves not only exists, but can bring about a profound change in their lives. The word God itself is repeated several times throughout the rest of the steps. This may present a problem for those individuals who are atheists or who have rejected the idea of God because of negative prior experiences with organized religion. (Others are comfortable from the outset with using the word God; it has no negative connotations for them.) Thinking of God as "Good Orderly Direction," rather than as the deity of a particular religion, helps skeptics, agnostics, and atheists, as well as those who still may have difficulty with the God of their childhood, to practice the steps and follow the program. Some members joke that GOD stands for "Group of Druggies" or "Group of Drunks."

› **God has no grandchildren.** Al-Anon/Nar-Anon slogan. When worried about the addiction of a grown child (or young adult), this slogan reminds members that each one of them is on his or her own journey, and that each one is capable of developing a relationship with God, who is considered by many to be a spiritual father. Even though a person is a son or daughter, he or she is nevertheless an autonomous person in the sight of God.

› **God is in the numbers.** Debtors Anonymous (DA) slogan. Vagueness about finances is one of the chief character defects of a compulsive debtor. So being told "God is in the numbers" may be frightening to a DA newcomer. It means that in order to find a higher power, a debtor must take an honest look at these numbers that are so frightening, especially when they total great sums of debt. However, the DA fellowship encourages and supports the newcomer to look clearly, forthrightly, and regularly at his or her financial records in order to work the steps of DA recovery.

› **Guilt is the gift that keeps on giving.** Guilt can be viewed as a gift when it provides a recovering person with the motivation to change. The fear or apprehension of feeling guilt can sometimes motivate an individual to continue to practice principles in all of his or her affairs. In that sense, guilt (like desperation) may often be a gift to a recovering person.

› **HALT(S): Hungry, Angry, Lonely, Tired, (being too Serious).** Any of these five states affecting one's physical mental, emotional, and spiritual well-being are believed to make a recovering individual vulnerable to relapse. Asking if someone in recovery is feeling any of these sensations or emotions is a quick way to evaluate whether it is time to put a "HALT(S)" to what he or she is doing, call his or her sponsor, and go to a meeting.

› **Higher-powered.** A play on the words "higher power," lightheartedly announcing that one is energized by a power higher or greater than oneself.

› **HOW it works.** Honesty, open-mindedness, and willingness are the keys to recovery.

› **I can't; we can.** The basis of the twelve-step program model is the healing benefits derived from one recovering individual helping another recovering individual. What one cannot accomplish alone, two or more can do together.

› *I'll* **drink poison to make** *you* **sick.** To cling to resentment against another does nothing to the other; instead it harms the person holding onto resentment. Holding onto resentments is usually why an individual will not go to a certain meeting or other fellowship gatherings/functions and this is dangerous because it can isolate and alienate the individual.

› **I may not be much, but I'm all I think about.** Self-deprecating humorous recognition by someone in recovery that he or she is being self-centered and/or self-obsessed. Regardless of how it manifests, addiction is all-consuming and those people who suffer from it are frequently only concerned with themselves while actively using. This self-centeredness does not simply vanish when the person stops using, drinking, or acting out a behavior. This expression is an ironic admission that an individual in recovery is aware of this defect.

› **If I don't change, my clean/sober/abstinent date will.** If a person who comes into recovery does not change his or her behavior and lifestyle, then he or she will most likely relapse. If he or she is lucky enough to make it back into the program, it will be with a new recovery date.

› **If you are in the center, it's harder to fall off the edge.** It is considered important to recovery and the recovery process to put oneself in the "middle of the herd," that is, in the middle of the recovery community. To stay on the edge of recovery or the recovery community puts one at risk of being vulnerable to using or returning to old behavior in difficult and/or challenging times. Think of animals who move in packs; those on the edges are at greater risk of being "picked off" by predators than those in the middle of the herd.

› **If you are too busy to pray, you are too busy.** People who make time to pray and center themselves usually find more peace and balance in recovery. A life in recovery that has no time in it for prayer may end in relapse. Making the time to pray and/or meditate adds value to all other activities.

› **If you do what you always did, you'll get what you always got.** The recovery process is all about change. The concept of doing something different does not just apply to someone who is new in recovery. There will be times when a person with long-term recovery is just not satisfied with what they are getting out of life or recovery. In such cases, it is important for that person to do something different (within the twelve-step program) if they want to get something different out of life.

› **If you don't have a home group, you are homeless.** A home group runs the meeting that a recovering person attends most frequently, where he or she has commitments, and at least some friends who will notice if he or she is absent, unhappy, or ill. Having a home group offers a life line for many people in recovery, making them feel a part of something and offering support when needed. Being accountable to one's home group is important; lack of accountability (not just to a home group) often leads to relapse for the recovering person.

› **If you don't pick up, you won't get loaded;** or **If you don't drink, you won't get drunk.** Members fear relapsing or reverting to an old behavior because for some, a relapse means certain death. While there are many things a recovering person must do for his or her recovery, the most important and primary action is to not use or act on addictive behaviors.

› **If you fail to change the person you were when you came in, that person will take you out.** The person who comes into a meeting for the first time is a person who only knows how to live life while using or acting out. That person does not have life skills to cope with the normal occurrences that can happen in life. The goal of the steps and recovery is to change, and if one does not change, he or she will ultimately relapse.

› **If you're still doing it, then it's not old behavior.** Persons in recovery distinguish between their "old," or diseased, behavior and their behavior in their new life in recovery. However, sometimes although one is in recovery, one's behavior is more appropriate to the "old" life.

› **I'm a puff away from a pack a day.** Nicotine Anonymous slogan that reminds members that even a puff can get the body caught up in craving cycles, and once that first puff is taken, the person cannot stop.

› **Insanity is doing the same thing over and over again, expecting different results.** While this saying is popular with those in twelve-step recovery, it is actually credited to Albert Einstein. It almost speaks for itself, but is particularly appropriate for the Second Step in recovery. If one expects to change, then he or she must take different actions from those that resulted in the problem. By taking different actions, an individual in recovery will give him- or herself the opportunity to experience a difference result.

› **Isolation: It's the darkroom where I develop my negatives.** A quip that encapsulates what happens to someone who isolates and remains aloof from others in the twelve-step fellowship who could offer him or her help; only negativity can ensue. Recovery cannot occur when an individual is acting alone or refusing assistance from others in recovery.

An isolated person tends to rely more and more heavily upon his or her character defects in order to cope with life. Dependence on defects is the "default position" of the person in order to fulfill his or her needs or wants; unfortunately, it often leads to relapse.

› **It Works!** or **It works if you work it!** A slogan affirming the idea that the twelve-step program is a success and people can and do recover—but only if they themselves work the program. (The words ". . . and you're worth it," are often added to these slogans and chanted at meetings after the closing prayer.)

› **It's hard to be grateful when you're hateful;** or **It's hard to be hateful when you're grateful.** Gratitude does not come naturally to people in active addiction who always want "more, more, more." But developing gratitude is a necessary component of twelve-step recovery. Being aware of when one is feeling "hateful" and replacing that feeling with gratitude helps recovering individuals maintain contact with their higher power and with the fellowship.

› **It's okay to visit the past, just don't bring a suitcase.** During a Fourth-Step inventory, a recovering person will need to review the past and write about his or her experiences, in order to take an honest self-assessment and make as thorough a house-cleaning as possible. But wallowing in guilt over past misdeeds is not helpful to the recovery process. The past is examined and past behaviors are noted in order that these behaviors may be avoided in the future. Past wrongs are noted in order that amends may be made; however, the past is not a stick that the recovering person uses to beat up him- or herself. Once the past is understood, it is put in its rightful place, and the individual moves on with recovery.

› **It's the first drink that gets you drunk.** AA slogan meaning that no alcoholic ever stops at one drink—the first drink leads to another, then another, and finally to complete intoxication.

> **Juggling is not balancing.** It's an understatement to say that people in recovery have a tendency to bite off more than they can chew. They will take on multiple projects or responsibilities, have difficulty saying no, and will spread themselves too thin especially when new to recovery. Juggling these projects is the opposite of maintaining a balanced life in recovery.

> **Just because you *have* a pain, doesn't mean you have to *be* one.** Walking through pain is challenging, even for a person with long-term recovery. The tendency for a recovering person who is in pain is to act out by lashing out at others. It is the goal of a recovering person to walk through emotional or physical pain by acknowledging feelings of discomfort, anger, sadness, etc. without lashing out at other people.

> **Just for today. (See also: One day at a time.)** A slogan in twelve-step programs used as a reminder for members that they only need to concentrate on not using or not acting out on a feeling with addictive behavior, in the present. Newcomers, especially, can become discouraged at the thought of abstaining for the rest of their lives, but the thought of doing so "just for today" is less daunting and feels more "doable."

Additionally, people in recovery have a tendency to project thoughts into the future or to dwell on memories and patterns of the past and this deprives them of living in the moment, which is where recovery actually occurs. Worry and frustration about potential outcomes robs individuals of life in the moment, prevents them from embracing recovery, and can often lead to destructive behavior in an attempt to control an outcome. Worry and fear often lead to relapse.

Just for Today is also the name of the daily meditation book of Narcotics Anonymous.

> **Keep coming back.** The Third Tradition says the only requirement of a twelve-step program is the desire to stop using, drinking, or acting out on a particular manifestation of addiction. If an individual relapses, his or her "membership" is not "revoked." The important thing is for him or her to get back to a meeting and start over again.

> **KISS.** Keep it simple, stupid. Refers to the tendency of some members to complicate or overanalyze the program when all that is required is to be honest, open-minded, and willing.

> **Learn to listen and listen to learn.** One of the hardest things for some newcomers to understand is that those who have been in recovery for a period of time do understand and can empathize with many of the feelings the new person is experiencing. The new person needs to hear what it is like to stay in recovery and work steps. The new person needs to listen to what he or she needs to do—the action he or she must take—in order to get another day clean/sober/abstinent. Recovery groups are not places for sharing all of one's feelings so much as they are for getting support in the action and steps that must be taken in order to stay in recovery.

> **Let go and let God.** A phrase that comes out of the Third Step, which calls for turning one's will over to a power greater than oneself. Many people in the program use the word God as a sort of shorthand for higher power, but they do not necessarily mean a traditional, religious concept of God. This slogan is merely advising the individual to stop worrying about matters he or she cannot control and accept that these things can and will work out, according to the will of God/a higher power.

> **Let go or get dragged.** Humorous variant of "let go and let God," expressing the idea that God's will *will* be done, whether one wants it or not, so the best attitude to take is one of acceptance.

> **Let it begin with me.** Al-Anon slogan taken from the last line of a circa 1955 hymn, "Let there be peace on earth . . . and let it begin with me." Indicates willingness to do the "next right thing" in spite of what others do, say, or think.

> **Letting go of the baggage.** In order to move forward in recovery, the recovering person must let go of those aspects from the past that do not serve him or her. These are often called resentments and must be addressed. This happens formally with a sponsor in the Fourth and

Fifth Steps. As people progress in recovery, "baggage" is picked up again, and they usually need to let go of this baggage regularly. The Tenth Step facilitates this process of letting go on a regular basis.

> **Life is painful. Misery is optional.** While it is virtually impossible to avoid pain—be it caused by the loss of a loved one, a relationship, financial security, or a job—the extent to which a person dwells in that pain is entirely up to him or her. Some of life's events are painful; it's one's emotional response that generates *misery*. Through regular step work, meeting attendance, and contact with a support group, a person can avoid being miserable, although no one has ever been able to avoid pain.

> **Live and let live.** Keep the focus on yourself and what needs to be changed in you in order for you to grow in recovery. Although others—in and out of recovery—may do things that trouble or annoy you, just live your life and let them live theirs.

> **Live in the solution.** The solution this phrase refers to is the Twelve Steps. Working and applying the Twelve Steps is a process that one must continue on a regular basis in order to face and solve life's problems. The steps are not an aspirin or a band-aid to be resorted to after the fact; they should be worked consistently and applied to the best of one's ability if a person's life is to improve.

> **Living life on life's terms.** The object of the game is to stay and live in recovery. This means not relapsing no matter what life throws at one. This may mean staying in recovery through the death of a loved one, divorce, the loss of jobs, or sometimes just simply a bad day or a string of bad days. It is not always the tragedies in life that can cause a relapse. Sometimes it is just going through life and becoming complacent about one's recovery, drifting away from meetings and others in recovery, and forgetting about the "basics of the program," which can and often does lead to a relapse.

› **Living the program.** To live the program means bringing what one learns in the program into every area of one's life. This saying ties back to several of the steps, including Steps Ten and Twelve: taking a regular personal inventory and practicing twelve-step principles in all of one's affairs helps one live in the program.

› **Look for the similarities, not the differences.** Newcomers often look for the ways they are different from other members they see in meetings. They may feel "I'm not *that* bad," or "If these people knew what I'd done, they'd reject me." Either of these thoughts keeps the newcomer separated and isolated. Looking for the similarities between fellowship members and themselves helps newcomers relate.

› **Meeting-makers make it.** Those who attend meetings regularly, in whatever twelve-step fellowship they belong, tend to have a higher success rate at staying in recovery. Meetings help form the basis of working a program.

› **Misery is optional.** Every life includes pain. It is the way one handles pain that makes the difference between bearable pain and (seemingly) unbearable misery.

› **My higher power has a first name, and it's not Will.** Most people in active addiction tried to run their lives on willpower, which naturally proved to be futile. No amount of willpower is enough to fight the disease of addiction. Turning one's will and life over to the care of a higher power is not easy, but it is easier than using willpower to get through difficulties.

› **Ninety meetings in ninety days; or 90-in-90.** Newcomers are encouraged to attend one twelve-step meeting every day for a period of at least ninety days. This enables the newcomer to meet people within his or her selected fellowship, as well as potential sponsors, become familiar with the program and the Twelve Steps, and to develop a new habit of attending meetings.

› *No* **is a complete sentence.** One of the most difficult things for many people in recovery is to set and maintain boundaries. Early in recovery an individual may feel that he or she needs to explain why he or she cannot spend time with someone who is still in active addiction. Simply saying "no" without an explanation is completely healthy, acceptable, and sufficient.

› **No major decisions in your first year.** A person entering recovery is on the brink of a new way of life. Removing drugs, alcohol, and addictive behaviors, while healthy and necessary, requires a great deal of adjustment and commitment. Without using, the recovering person is now swamped with new sensations—feelings and emotions masked by active addiction must now be processed in a natural and healthy way. Additional stresses, like changing jobs, relationship partners, or homes can be too overwhelming during the first year. Newcomers to recovery often feel a surge of energy and purposefulness, but it's best to use those impulses to concentrate on building the foundation that can support their new lives in recovery.

Embarking on new relationships, careers, etc., may provide a euphoric distraction from the difficult work of staying in recovery and may derail an individual's efforts to do so.

› **No matter what your past, you have a spotless future.** The past is the past, and cannot be changed, but the future lies ahead, unblemished. Following a program of recovery can help it stay that way.

› **Nothing tastes as good as abstinence.** Overeaters Anonymous slogan; please note—abstinence in OA does not (and cannot) mean complete abstinence from food—it means abstaining from compulsive food behaviors.

› **One day at a time. (See also: Just for today.)** This slogan expresses the truth underpinning all twelve-step programs; that all one can do is stay clean/sober/abstinent in the present moment. The old timer with twenty-four years is no more clean/sober/abstinent than the newcomer with twenty-four hours; each one is in recovery *today*; each could relapse tomorrow. This is the basis of much of the philosophy of acceptance, humility, honesty, tolerance, and willingness that is found in twelve-step recovery.

› **People who don't go to meetings don't hear about what happens to people who don't go to meetings.** In meetings, it's not uncommon to hear from a new person who is coming back from a relapse. More often than not that person will share about what happened before the relapse, e.g., he or she was not going to meetings or not calling his or her sponsor or not working the steps. People who are not at the meeting never get the chance or opportunity to hear from the people who are suffering as a result of not doing the simple, fundamental things that help one to stay in recovery.

› **Plan plans, not results.** Regardless of the "one day at a time" or "just for today" philosophy that is key to staying in recovery, over time, a recovering person will likely become successful at making and keeping plans. This is fine as long as he or she realizes that plans have a way of working out differently than he or she wishes. Disappointment can lead to relapse if one is not spiritually fit.

› **Principles before personalities.** From the Twelfth Tradition, the idea is to practice the spiritual principles learned through working the Twelve Steps regardless of the people involved. The practice of putting principles ahead of any personal differences ensures that regardless of the people (personalities) involved in any situation, the recovering person practices the concepts learned through working the steps.

› **Procrastination is fear in five syllables.** People in recovery sometimes put off doing something (like making amends) because of fear—fear of losing control of the outcome, fear of failure, or even fear of success.

> **Projection—living in the wreckage of the future.** Most people can become overwhelmed by thinking about the future, particularly in early recovery. One must live in the present day, based on what is happening during that day and leave the results to a higher power or the process of recovery, doing the daily footwork to stay in recovery regardless of what happens in the future, without reservations.

> **Put your recovery first and everything else in your life will be first-rate.** Make recovery your daily priority and your life will improve in all ways.

> **Quick doesn't stick; or Recovery is a journey, not a destination. (See also: Easy does it; and Recovery is a process, not an event.)** Most individuals in active addiction are almost always more interested in instant gratification than in working for lasting change. The disease of addiction is the disease of "more is not enough" and "instant gratification takes too long." Impatience bedevils those suffering with addiction, and the time required to work on recovery can seem impossibly long for those who are used to changing their feelings in the time it takes to swallow a pill or a drink, or to eat a donut, or pull the lever on a slot machine. It is important to remember that the Twelve Steps will change one's life, but will do so slowly.

> **Recovery is an action word.** This is said to imply that recovery means actually doing things such as getting and using a sponsor to work the Twelve Steps, attending meetings, reaching out to others in recovery, and sponsoring other members of the program an individual attends. Recovery is not simply a thing or state of mind that an individual is in, but instead, is something that a person must practice regularly in order to maintain freedom from active addiction.

> **Regardless of . . . .** Just as addiction can happen to anyone, recovery can happen for anyone—believer or nonbeliever, old or young, gay or straight, married or single, educated or uneducated, jobless or employed, rich or poor, or any combination thereof. And a person in recovery can remain in recovery, regardless of any circumstance or misfortune.

> **Rule 62. (See also: Take the program seriously . . . .)** AA-related slogan that encourages members to not take themselves so seriously.

> **Serenity precedes prosperity.** Debtors Anonymous slogan. Expresses the idea, common to all twelve-step fellowships, that spiritual fitness must be sought before material fitness, but that if one seeks spirituality and serenity, material security will follow.

> **Show up to grow up.** One must "show up" for meetings, service commitments, commitments with one's friends, employer, or sponsor, and oneself through doing step work if recovery is to succeed.

> **Stay away from the first bet.** Gamblers Anonymous slogan, comparable to the suggestion (in various forms) found in most twelve-step fellowships to stay away from the first of whatever manifestation of addiction over which a person is powerless.

> **Stick with the winners.** Who are the winners? The ones who are successful in recovery. This doesn't mean materially, but spiritually. Winners are the ones who are living a good and worthwhile life in recovery. These are usually the people who show up for meetings, who work steps, who are of service in the program, and who are good examples of how recovery works in a person's life.

> **Surrender to win.** Surrender is a key principle of the First Step. Part one of the step is acceptance of the disease of addiction or surrendering to the idea that one is powerless over the disease of addiction. Part two of that step is continual surrender by not using or acting on a behavior, and instead, focusing on taking action in recovery.

> **Take the program seriously, not yourself. (See also: Rule 62.)** A benefit of recovery is the ability to laugh at oneself or difficult situations because the recovering person knows that he or she is not in control, and is only responsible for doing "the footwork."

Although addiction is a chronic, progressive, and potentially fatal disease, in recovery there is much laughter among fellowship members—to the annoyance of some, who feel that such a serious disease should only be discussed in serious terms. However, there are those who believe that the laughter heard in the rooms of recovery is actually caused by identification with the situations that fellowship members recount in their sharing, and as such is very much in line with the twelve-step mandate that says recovery comes when one person in recovery talks to another.

> **Take what you need and leave the rest.** Much of the language and philosophy of twelve-step recovery is strange and perplexing to the newcomer. The advice to "take what you need and leave the rest," means to embrace what makes sense to one and set the rest aside. The newcomer may come back to it with greater understanding when he or she has more recovery time in the program.

Additionally, a newcomer to meetings may notice that because of the freedom to share "from the heart," some things are shared that are puzzling, odd, or downright obnoxious. Some people do take advantage of this opportunity to have the undivided attention of the group, and instead of sharing about the recovery process, working the steps, or their experiences, they want to talk about their day or go into some detail about something that others really do not want to hear. They may be insulting or insensitive to others in the room. Others may feel the need or desire to share directly "at" another or give advice or feedback directly to another member and engage in "cross-talk," which is generally frowned upon. This slogan suggests that one leaves or disregards the odd or bizarre things occasionally heard at meetings, and carry home the words that make the most sense.

> **Take your own inventory.** From the Fourth Step, which calls for a "searching and fearless moral inventory" of one's self. One should look at his or her own behaviors, rather than judge others for theirs. Looking at the character defects of others will not help a person work on his or her character defects.

› **Taking responsibility for my own recovery.** Recovery is a personal process; no one else can "make" another person recover. Friends and family would have done it by now if it were possible. A person in recovery must take responsibility for attending meetings, finding and working with a sponsor, meeting commitments, and working the steps.

› **Talking out of the side of your neck.** Futile or fruitless, worthless talk. May also mean lying or speaking about things that one does not fully understand or have sufficient information to speak about. This is often done in an effort to appear knowledgeable or important.

› **Terminally unique/terminal uniqueness.** A feeling that one is different from another. This is common among many individuals in recovery. The fatal illness of addiction will progress to its inevitable outcome if not checked by the process of recovery, which begins when one person in recovery shares with another person in recovery and both realize that neither one of them is "unique."

› **The elevator is broken. Use the steps.** There is no easy way to recover. The process of recovery is simple, but it requires work. Those who suffer from addiction are usually looking for instant gratification or an "elevator," rather than doing the work necessary in the "steps," otherwise known as the Twelve Steps.

› **The gifts of the program can take us out of the program.** A popular recovery saying indicating that life in recovery can become so good that one may become "too busy," or feel "too cured" to attend meetings, meet service commitments, write or otherwise work the steps, etc. These omissions are all indicators that a person is most likely on the road to relapse. One must always remember that unless recovery comes first, the "gifts of recovery" will not last.

› **The nature of recovery.** The nature of recovery is the process of working the steps and practicing spiritual principles such as compassion, tolerance, acceptance, honesty, open-mindedness, and willingness.

› **The next indicated step (or taking the next right step).** Rather than focusing on the rest of one's life or major choices that might need to be made, a recovering person may be better served by just focusing on what he or she needs to do next.

› **The outsides don't match the insides.** The "outside" of someone's life could look really good, but he or she may be falling apart on the inside because of not taking care of the things he or she needs to be taking care of, such as working steps, attending meetings, doing service work, etc. Likewise, things may appear to be falling apart on the outside for a person, but if his or her program is intact and robust, then that is what is important.

› **The road gets narrower.** The idea of the "road getting narrower" is an often-heard term in many twelve-step meetings, and refers to the metaphorical road that one travels along in recovery. It is said to mean that as one continues on the path of recovery, old behaviors that were once acceptable may need to be discarded. Lying, cheating, stealing, cruelty, intolerance, etc. are no longer options; as the "road" narrows, these practices no longer fit. As a person becomes more focused on his or her recovery, the ways that person can "act out" are far more limited. Without over-interpreting this saying, some believe that the road getting narrower implies that one has fewer ways of acting on addiction the longer he or she stays in recovery, but that one's opportunities for growth and life actually grow wider.

› **The rooms/these rooms.** The meeting rooms where twelve-step program meetings are held.

› **The steps are the answer;** or **The answer is in the steps.** When a member is confused about a right course of action, rather than listen to another member who may be more than willing to dole out advice, the member would be better served by remembering that the program is based on the Twelve Steps, and within the steps is usually a right and safe approach to any question or problem. Working the steps with a sponsor will help members cope with "life on life's terms."

Every problem life presents has been addressed in most twelve-step programs, and though the programs are not designed to answer all of life's questions, they provide a framework that allows the individual members to accept "life on life's terms" and remain in recovery.

> **The steps keep us from suicide; the traditions, from homicide.** A humorous reminder that the steps are considered a personal process, helping a person in recovery to build and heal his or her relationship with him- or herself. The traditions, while written in relation to the group or fellowship, have often been studied by individuals who view them as guidelines for helping to carry the message of recovery to those still suffering from addiction.

> **The three most dangerous words for a person in recovery: "I've been thinking."** Recognizes that the thinking of an individual in recovery has not, in many instances in the past, resulted in safe or sane decision-making. A lighthearted reminder to the newcomer to discuss any new ideas or projects with a sponsor or friends who have more time in recovery, at least until he or she has had the opportunity to work through the Twelve Steps. After a person has been in recovery for a period of time and worked the steps, he or she can begin to trust his or her thinking to a larger degree.

> **The war is over and you lost.** A friendly reminder that one's addiction is always going to be stronger than oneself, and that the only way to "win" is to surrender. Sometimes said to a newcomer who may be trying to justify his or her continued using or acting on addictive behavior and to prompt the person to accept that he or she can no longer continue to use or act out.

> **Time takes time.** It's natural to want to have the degree of serenity that is often seen among some old timers and others who are in long-term recovery. It's important to remember that they were newcomers once, and it took time as well as adherence to the program for them to reach the point they are at today. Anyone who has the desire to get better can also attain this kind of time by working the program of recovery.

› **Today is a gift; that's why it's called the present.** Every day that someone with addiction stays in recovery is a successful day.

› **Trying is dying.** This saying came from the idea that many people in recovery will use the word "try" as an excuse for not doing something. They may say they will *try* to work the steps, *try* to call their sponsor, or *try* to remain abstinent, and the response from another recovering member may be "trying is dying," because someone in recovery simply needs to commit to *doing* that thing he or she is actually resisting doing. To say that one is "trying" is often a copout, excuse, or reservation in one's program.

› **Turn it over.** In the Third Step, the recovering person is asked to turn his or her will over to a power greater than him- or herself. The process of "turning it over" means to practice the program principles of trust and faith, instead of acting out in destructive behaviors. This can also be accomplished through prayer and meditation. The act of surrendering a situation, person, etc. to the care of a loving higher power.

› **Walking the talk; or Walk the walk, don't just talk the talk;** or **Watch your feet.** What people say in meetings is meaningless unless their "talk" is matched with their "walk"; that is, unless they practice the principles of the program outside the meeting, with others in and out of the program, to the best of their ability on a daily basis.

› **We grow up in public.** The process of recovery is a "public" process in that one must reveal him- or herself—in a general way in meetings with other recovering people and in a specific way with a sponsor. It is also a process that teaches to many the things they should have learned as they were growing up had they not begun to live in their disease. These things include how to be a friend, a parent, an employee, etc. As people learn and grow in the group, many feel they are "growing up" in public.

› **Whatever I obsess about becomes my higher power. Do I want money problems as my higher power?** Debtors Anonymous slogan. Worry and anxiety about one's problems, financial or otherwise, cannot solve one's problems. Working the steps, helping another, "cleaning up one's own side of the street," prayer and meditation—these are the kinds of things that lead one to a conscious contact with a higher power. It's generally observed in most twelve-step fellowships that the person or thing one thinks about the most can be considered that person's higher power; where it once was a manifestation of the person's addiction, the person can now choose a higher power of his or her own understanding and start to heal.

› **When all else fails, follow directions.** Refers to the tendency of some newcomers to resist following their sponsors' suggestions/instructions until they are in emotional pain or suffering from some other kinds of consequences.

› **When the pain of staying the same is greater than the fear of change, we'll change.** The fear of the unknown is often greater than the pain of the familiar; however, once the pain of the familiar becomes great enough, a person will stop and face the fear of what the new action may offer.

› **Where-and-when.** A term used for a schedule of recovery meetings in a particular area; also known as a meeting list. The meeting lists for local meetings, which are usually updated regularly, contains information such as meeting location, address, meeting time, meeting classification, (whether the meeting is open, closed, a literature study, speaker meeting, etc.), whether the meeting is smoking/non-smoking, or handicapped-accessible. Planning which meetings to attend is helpful to newcomers and helps them to take responsibility for their recovery.

› **Would you rather be right or happy?** It's difficult for someone new to recovery, or most any person, to admit that he or she was/is wrong. To admit that one is wrong frees one from having to cling to a posture of righteousness and enables one to embrace a different path. This is also a reference to being open-minded, a key principle to working the Second Step.

› **Yesterday is history, tomorrow a mystery.** The only thing a recovering person can do about the past is work a program of recovery today. Even making amends for past wrongs requires working a program in the here-and-now. One does not know what will happen in the future, so all a recovering person can do is focus on what he or she can do for his or her recovery each day.

› **Yets.** Things a person has not done up to a given point in time. The idea that although a particular situation or event, e.g., divorce, a prison term, loss of children, etc., has not occurred in someone's life due to his or her addiction, it is possible it could happen in the future should they relapse.

In sharing at a meeting, people may say of something, "That is one of my *yets*." Admitting one has yets is admitting that while one has not plumbed the absolute depths of degradation, it could happen yet, if one were to relapse. Could contribute to reservations, e.g., "I never prostituted myself for drugs; maybe I'm not a *real addict*," or "I never got a DUI, maybe I'm not a *real alcoholic*."

› **You are a member when you say you are.** There is no application process nor are there dues or fees for twelve-step program membership. The only requirement is a desire to stop using/drinking/overeating/gambling/compulsive spending/etc.

› **You cannot be in fear and faith at the same time.** Living in faith means trusting that all will be well; living in fear means dreading that all will be ill. All human beings, not just those in recovery, experience fear; it's a natural and sometimes useful part of life that helps one avoid dangers. But for people with the disease of addiction, living in fear is part of their addictive behavior; trying to evade those fears led them to the escapism of using/drinking/acting out/etc.

The attributes of fear and faith are at odds; one cannot act on fear-based addictive thinking or take character-defect-based actions and at the same time act in faith, recovery-oriented, spiritual-principle-based actions. This slogan is often misinterpreted or misrepresented to make one believe that he or she cannot feel fear or faith at the same time. However, one of the first things a newcomer learns in recovery is that just because a person feels, desires, or has a thought to perform a certain action he or she is not bound to perform that action, i.e., one can be afraid of using drugs—a healthy fear—but one does not need to use nor does that mean that person's recovery is in danger.

> **You can't get indigestion from swallowing your pride.** It is often humbling to admit that one has been acting out in his or her disease, that he or she is powerless, or that his or her behavior has been based in his or her disease. But admitting these things, or "swallowing one's pride," is necessary if one is to become open-minded to taking different actions. If one is to do a thorough Eighth or Ninth Step, it will be necessary to set aside pride and admit prior wrongs, in order to get the relief promised by the program.

> **You can't save your face and your ass at the same time.** Recovering people who try to maintain the appearance or illusion of having a manageable life run the risk of relapse. A person in recovery must accept and admit powerlessness and unmanageability in those areas he or she wishes to change in order to recover. It is also necessary, when a person in recovery is in pain or needs help, to reach out to others and admit that he or she is in pain.

re·cov·er·y |ri'kəvərē|

How to Find Meetings

You can check the websites or phone numbers of the program you are interested in for the most up-to-date information before contacting any of the locations or addresses listed below. If the number is no longer valid you can also contact directory assistance in your local area. Most twelve-step programs also have local helpline numbers that you can obtain through contacting directory assistance or by looking in a phone book. Your doctor or clergyperson may also be able to refer you.

It is very important to know that none of these phone numbers is a crisis hotline. In most cases the phones are either answered by volunteers or employees (special workers) who are not, in any case, professional counselors. For emergencies, always call 9-1-1 or the local emergency number in your area.

ADULT CHILDREN OF ALCOHOLICS
Adult Children of Alcoholics WSO
PO Box 3216
Torrance, CA 90510
(562) 595-7831
www.adultchildren.org

AL-ANON and ALATEEN
Al-Anon Family Group Headquarters, Inc.
1600 Corporate Landing Parkway
Virginia Beach, VA 23454-5617
(757) 563-1600
www.al-anon.alateen.org

ALCOHOLICS ANONYMOUS

General Service Office
AA World Services, Inc.
PO Box 459
New York, NY 10163
(212) 870-3400
www.aa.org

ANOREXICS AND BULIMICS ANONYMOUS

Anorexics and Bulimics Anonymous
Main PO Box 125
Edmonton, AB T5J 2G9
Canada
(780) 443-6077
www.anorexicsandbulimicsanonymous.com

CRYSTAL METH ANONYMOUS (CMA)

Crystal Meth Anonymous General Services
4470 W. Sunset Blvd.
Suite 107, PMB 555
Los Angeles, CA 90027-6302
(213) 488-4455
www.crystalmeth.org

CLUTTERERS ANONYMOUS

Clutterers Anonymous WSO
PO Box 91413
Los Angeles, CA 90009-1413\
(310) 281-6064 (Recorded Meeting List)
www.clutterersanonymous.net

COCAINE ANONYMOUS

Cocaine Anonymous WSO
PO Box 492000
Los Angeles, CA 90049-8000
(310) 559-5833
www.ca.org

CODEPENDENTS ANONYMOUS

CoDA, Fellowship Services Office
P.O. Box 33577
Phoenix, AZ 85067-3577
(602) 277-7991
www.coda.org

CODEPENDENTS OF SEX ADDICTS

International Service Office of Codependents of Sex Addicts (COSA)
PO Box 14537
Minneapolis, MN 55414
(763) 537-6904
www.cosa-recovery.org

DEBTORS ANONYMOUS

General Service Office
PO Box 920888
Needham, MA 02492-0009
(800) 421-2383
www.debtorsanonymous.org

DEPRESSED ANONYMOUS

PO Box 17414
Louisville, KY 40217
(502) 569-1989
www.depressedanon.com

DUAL RECOVERY ANONYMOUS

Dual Recovery Anonymous
World Network Central Office
PO Box 8107
Prairie Village, KS 66208
(913) 991-2703 (9 am–5 pm Central Time-Leave Message for Callback)
http://draonline.org

EMOTIONS ANONYMOUS

Emotions Anonymous International
PO Box 4245
St. Paul, MN 55104-0245
(651) 647-9712
www.emotionsanonymous.org

FAMILIES ANONYMOUS

Families Anonymous
PO Box 3475
Culver City, CA 90231-3475
(800) 736-9805
www.familiesanonymous.org

FOOD ADDICTS ANONYMOUS

Food Addicts Anonymous
World Service Office
529 N W Prima Vista Blvd.
#301A
Port St. Lucie, FL 34983
(561) 967-3871
www.foodaddictsanonymous.org

GAM-ANON

Gam-Anon International Service Office, Inc.
PO Box 157
Whitestone, NY 11357
(718) 352-1671
www.gam-anon-org

GAMBLERS ANONYMOUS

International Service Office
PO Box 17173
Los Angeles, CA 90017
(213) 386-8789
www.gamblersanonymous.org

MARIJUANA ANONYMOUS

Marijuana Anonymous World Services
PO Box 2912
Van Nuys, CA 91404
(800) 766-6779
www.marijuana-anonymous.org

NARCOTICS ANONYMOUS

NA World Services, Inc.
PO Box 9999
Van Nuys, California 91409 USA
(818) 773-9999
www.na.org

NICOTINE ANONYMOUS

Nicotine Anonymous World Services
419 Main Street
PMB #370
Huntington Beach, CA 92648
(877) 879-6422
www.nicotine-anonymous.org

ON-LINE GAMERS ANONYMOUS

On-Line Gamers Anonymous World Services
104 Miller Lane
Harrisburg, PA 17110
(612) 245-1115
www.olganon.org

OVEREATERS ANONYMOUS

Overeaters Anonymous World Service Office
PO Box 44020
Rio Rancho, NM 87174-4020
(505) 891-2664
www.oa.org

SEX ADDICTS ANONYMOUS

International Service Office of SAA
PO Box 70949
Houston, TX 77270
(713) 869-4902
www.sexaa.org

SEXAHOLICS ANONYMOUS

Sexaholics Anonymous International Central Office
PO Box 3565
Brentwood, TN 37024
(866) 424-8777
www.sa.org

SEX AND LOVE ADDICTS ANONYMOUS

Fellowship-Wide Services Office
1550 NE Loop 410, Ste 118
San Antonio, TX 78209
(210) 828-7900
www.slaafws.org

SEXUAL COMPULSIVES ANONYMOUS

Sexual Compulsives Anonymous
PO Box 1585, Old Chelsea Station
New York, NY 10011
(800) 977-4325
www.sca-recovery.org

SEX WORKERS ANONYMOUS

Sex Workers Anonymous
PO Box 3535
Tonopah, NV 89049
(775) 482-8756
www.sexworkersanonymous.com

WORKAHOLICS ANONYMOUS
World Service Organization
PO Box 289
Menlo Park, CA 94026-0289
(510) 273-9253
www.workaholics-anonymous.org

Available from Central Recovery Press
www.centralrecoverypress.com

PAIN RECOVERY

A Day without Pain
Mel Pohl, MD, FASAM • ISBN-13: 978-0-9799869-5-6 • $14.95 US

Pain Recovery: How to Find Balance and Reduce Suffering from Chronic Pain
Mel Pohl, MD, FASAM; Frank J. Szabo, Jr., LADC; Dan Shiode, Ph.D.; Rob Hunter, Ph.D. • ISBN-13: 978-0-9799869-9-4 • $20.95 US

Pain Recovery for Families: How to Find Balance When Someone Else's Chronic Pain Becomes Your Problem Too
Mel Pohl, MD, FASAM; Frank J. Szabo, Jr., LADC; Dan Shiode, Ph.D.; Rob Hunter, Ph.D. • ISBN-13: 978-0-9818482-3-5 • $20.95 US

Meditations for Pain Recovery
Tony Greco • ISBN 13: 978-0-9818482-8-0 • $16.95 US

INSPIRATIONAL

Guide Me in My Recovery: Prayers for Times of Joy and Times of Trial
The Reverend John T. Farrell, Ph.D.
ISBN-13: 978-1-936290-00-0 • $12.95 US

Special hardcover gift edition:
ISBN-13: 978-1-936290-02-4 • $19.95 US

The Soul Workout: Getting and Staying Spiritually Fit
Helen H. Moore • ISBN-13: 978-0-9799869-8-7 • $12.95 US

Tails of Recovery: Addicts and the Pets That Love Them
Nancy A. Schenck • ISBN-13: 978-0-9799869-6-3 • $19.95 US

Of Character: Building Assets in Recovery
Denise D. Crosson, Ph.D. • ISBN-13: 978-0-9799869-2-5 • $12.95 US

MEMOIRS

Leave the Light On: A Memoir of Recovery and Self-Discovery
Jennifer Storm • ISBN-13: 978-0-9818482-2-8 • $14.95 US

The Mindful Addict: A Memoir of the Awakening of a Spirit
Tom Catton • ISBN-13: 978-0-9818482-7-3 • $18.95 US

Becoming Normal: An Ever-Changing Perspective
Mark Edick • ISBN-13: 978-0-9818482-1-1 • $14.95 US

YOUNG ADULT AND YOUNG READER

First Star I See
Jaye Andras Caffrey, illustrated by Lynne Adamson
ISBN-13: 978-1-936290-01-7 • $12.95 US

The Secret of Willow Ridge: Gabe's Dad Finds Recovery
Helen H. Moore, illustrated by John Blackford
Foreword by Claudia Black, Ph.D.
ISBN-13: 978-0-9818482-0-4 • $12.95 US

Mommy's Gone to Treatment
Denise D. Crosson, Ph.D., illustrated by Mike Motz
ISBN-13: 978-0-9799869-1-8 • $14.95 US

Mommy's Coming Home from Treatment
ISBN-13: 978-0-9799869-4-9 • $14.95 US

RELATIONSHIPS

*From Heartbreak to Heart's Desire: Developing a Healthy GPS
(Guy Picking System)*
Dawn Maslar, MS • ISBN-13: 978-0-9818482-6-6 • $14.95 US

Disentangle: When You've Lost Your Self in Someone Else
Nancy L. Johnston, MS, LPC, LSATP
ISBN-13: 978-1-936290-03-1 • $15.95 US

JOURNALS

*My First Year in Recovery: A Journal for the Journey
(Second Edition)*
The Editors of Central Recovery Press
ISBN-13: 978-0-9818482-4-2 • $19.95 US

*My Five-Year Recovery Planner: Looking to the Future,
One Day at a Time*
The Editors of Central Recovery Press
ISBN-13: 978-0-9818482-9-7 • $19.95 US

My Pain Recovery Journal
The Editors of Central Recovery Press
ISBN-13: 978-0-9799869-7-0 • $17.95 US